Based on CET 2012 (MCI)

Multiple Choice Questions in Dermatology

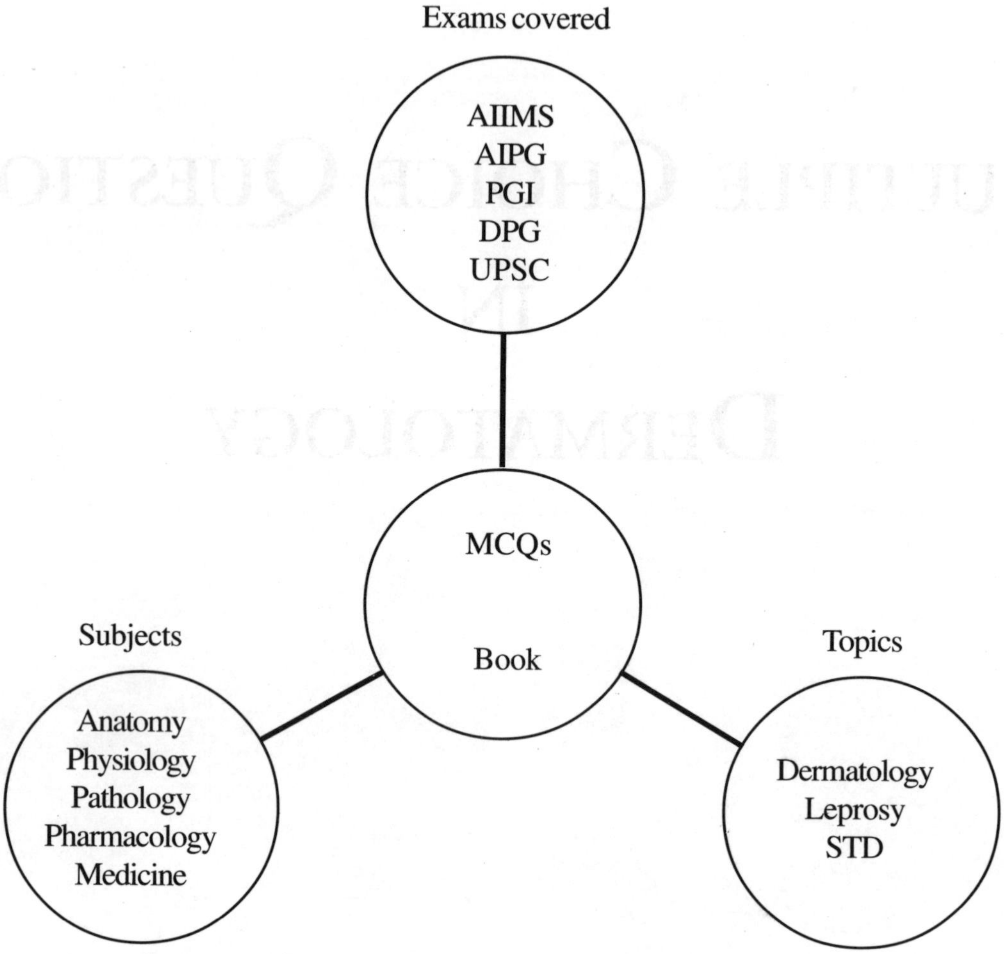
Exams covered
AIIMS
AIPG
PGI
DPG
UPSC
MCQs
Book
Subjects
Anatomy
Physiology
Pathology
Pharmacology
Medicine
Topics
Dermatology
Leprosy
STD

Multiple Choice Questions in Dermatology

(Based on Standard Textbooks of Dermatology)

Editors

DR KABIR SARDANA
MD, DNB, MNAMS
Associate Professor and Nodal Officer STD
Maulana Azad Medical College and Lok Nayak Hospital
New Delhi

DR VIJAY K GARG
MD, MNAMS
Director-Professor and Head of the Department
Department of Dermatology
Maulana Azad Medical College
New Delhi

PEEPEE
PUBLISHERS AND DISTRIBUTORS (P) LTD.

MCQs in Dermatology

Published by
Pawaninder P. Vij

Peepee Publishers and Distributors (P) Ltd.
Head Office: 160, Shakti Vihar, Pitam Pura, Delhi-110 034 (India)

Correspondence Address:

7/31, First Floor, Ansari Road, Daryaganj, Post Box-7243
New Delhi-110 002 (India)

Ph: 65195868, 9811156083, 23246245

e-mail: peepee160@yahoo.co.in

e-mail: peepee160@rediffmail.com

e-mail: peepee160@gmail.com

www.peepeepub.com

First Edition: 2010
Second Edition: 2011

ISBN: 978 81 8445 102 3

I dedicate this book to my parents ….

Major General KN Sardana – the most hardworking, honest person I have known….
My mother Amba Sardana who in these times also has faith in God ….

My wife Dr Supriya who is the wind beneath my wings and the bedrock of my life....

My daughter Zoya …. the light of our lives ….

All the students who have contributed and still do ….

And the Medical Examination system in our country which examines students by written examinations and viva while they are pursuing their MBBS

But ….

Sets papers based on MCQs when they take entrance exams….

For students

Be good, the best in what you do
There is respect for a good teacher of Anatomy, Biochemistry, Physiology
Or
Medicine, Surgery, Radiology….

Just be the best in what you do….

And be honest about it ….

Not everyone gets Radiology or Dermatology
It's good because we need more good doctors
Not superspecialists !

"Gayatri Mantra"

गायत्री मंत्र

ॐ भूर्भुवः स्वः
तत्सवितुर्वरेण्यम्
भर्गो देवस्य धीमहि
धियो यो नः प्रचोदयात्।

"OM BHUR, OM BHUVAHA, OM SWAHA, OM MAHAHA, OM JANAHA, OM TAPAHA, OM SATYAM, OM TAT SAVITUR VARENYAM BHARGHO DEVASYA DHIMAHI DHIYO YONAHA PRACHODAYAT."

"O God, You are the giver of life, the remover of pain and sorrow, the bestower of happiness; O Creator of the Universe, may we receive Your supreme sin-destroying light; may You guide our intellect in the right direction."

KARAMDHARMA

Bhagavad-gita (4.17-18)

One who sees inaction in action, and action in inaction, is intelligent among men, and he is in the transcendental position, although engaged in all sorts of activities.

Endowed with wisdom, giving up the fruits resulting from actions, attaining self-realization and freed from the bondage of birth, verily they go to that abode which is free from evil.

Established in yoga, O Dhananjaya (Arjuna), perform actions, giving up attachment, and unconcerned as to the success or failure.

To work alone you have the right, but never claim its results. Let not the result of actions be your motive, nor be attached to inaction.

Not by mere abstaining from action does a man reach the state of actionlessness, nor by mere renunciation does he arrive at perfection.

PREFACE

After 2 years of the first edition and multiple feedbacks we have done the following changes:

- Papers of the last 2 years of the major exams have been discussed first with detailed explanations.
- Almost 40-60% of MCQs are from the MCQs book and 100% from the textbook….
- The first edition was so successful that a reprint had to be ordered.
- Based on the success of the first edition the second edition is out with more controversial questions from various exams.

I would like to thank Mr Vij and his team including Pawan Sharma who worked on this edition in a record time…

We have added a special section on the MCI guidelines for exams also.

Please feel free to contribute and ask MCQ…

Dr Kabir Sardana

Kabir_sardana1@rediffmail.com

EDITORS

DR KABIR SARDANA
MD, DNB, MNAMS
Associate Professor
Maulana Azad Medical College and Lok Nayak Hospital
New Delhi

DR VIJAY K GARG
MD, MNAMS
Director-Professor and Head
Maulana Azad Medical College and Lok Nayak Hospital
New Delhi

MAIN CONTRIBUTORS

Dr Kabir Sardana
MD, DNB, MNAMS
Associate Professor
Maulana Azad Medical College and Lok Nayak Hospital
Delhi

Dr Anjali Madan
MBBS (Lady Hardinge Medical College)
DPG 12, 2nd Year PG
Maulana Azad Medical College and Lok Nayak Hospital
Delhi

Dr Pooja Agarwal
MBBS (KGMC, Lucknow)
AIPG 43, 2nd Year PG
Maulana Azad Medical College and Lok Nayak Hospital
Delhi

Dr Shrinkhala Khanna
MBBS (Maulana Azad Medical College)
DPG 9, AIPG 74
2nd Year PG
Maulana Azad Medical College and Lok Nayak Hospital
Delhi

Dr Rakesh
1st Year PG
Anesthesia
UCMS and GTB Hospital
Delhi

OTHERS....

Dr Khushboo
MD
AIPG 25, DPG Rank 30
Senior Resident
Maulana Azad Medical College and Lok Nayak Hospital
Delhi

Dr Shuchi
MD
AIPG 66, DPG Rank 4
Senior Resident
Maulana Azad Medical College and Lok Nayak Hospital
Delhi

Dr Chitra
MBBS
(Maulana Azad Medical College)
3rd Year PG
Maulana Azad Medical College and Lok Nayak Hospital
Delhi

Dr Mukesh
MBBS (University College of Medical Sciences)
3rd Year PG
Maulana Azad Medical College and Lok Nayak Hospital
Delhi

How to use the book?

The book can be used by either students who also have the textbook (preferable) or those who do not have the textbook. A brief using pattern is suggested.

Chapter	*Comprehensive Textbook of DermatologyΩ*	*Stand alone*
I. MCQs of 2009-11	Detailed Explanations are given	
II. Chapter-wise MCQs	The MCQs are based on the chapter of the book	These are *tough MCQs* of AIIMS/PGI/ DPG standards. You can read the book you have but most likely you will require to read standard guidelines and professional books of dermatology for answers
III. Exam based MCQs Section-wise (Based on actual exams held for last 10 years)	All the answers are based on the book	The MCQs are quick revision and placed topic-wise. Important MCQs are marked
IV. Controversial MCQs	Explanations are given in the MCQs book	Explanations are given in the MCQs book
V. Exam Papers AIPG/AIIMS	All the answers are already given in the book	100% accurate answers Better than guide books
VI. Test Series	One line easy answers are given of tough MCQ	One line easy answers are given of tough MCQ

Note:

Ω Those who have the book can read it as an addendum to his book and most of the MCQs are marked in bold in the text book.
Explanation given in the book.

AIIMS	Section 1, 2, 3, Relevant papers, Section 4, 6
AIPG	Section 1, 3, Relevant papers, Section 4, 6
DPG	Section 1, 3, Relevant papers, Section 4, 6
UPSC	Section 1, 2, 3, Relevant papers, Section 4, 6
State Exams	Section 1, 2, 3, Relevant papers, Section 4, 6
Rapid Reading	Section 1, 3, Section 4, 6
CET Mock Test	To be done if CET is notified by MCI.

UPDATE ON MCI RECOMMENDATIONS

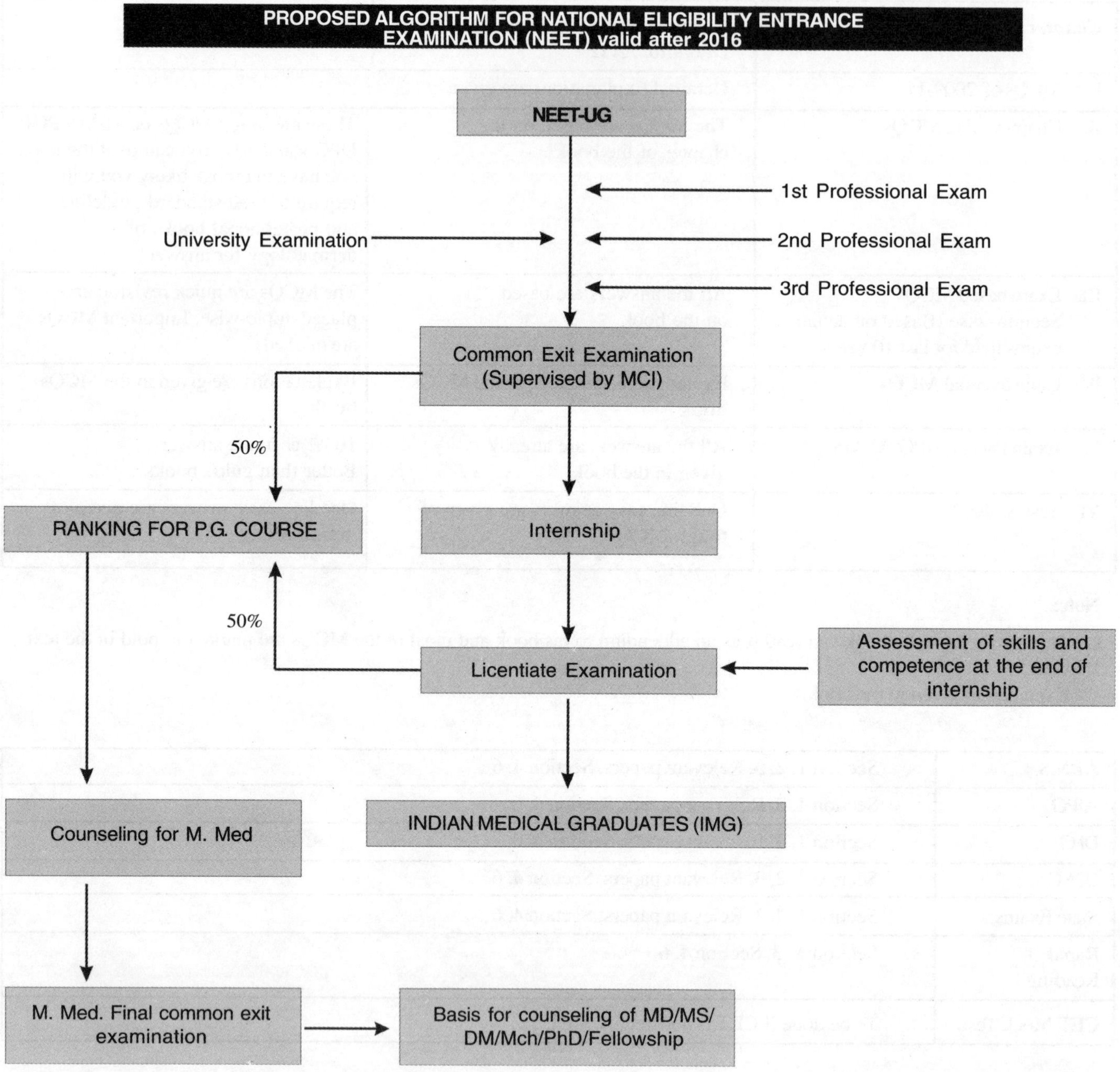

Note: 1. NEET–National Eligibility Entrance Test.
2. This plan would be valid after year 2016.

SUGGESTED ALGORITHM FOR PG COURSE

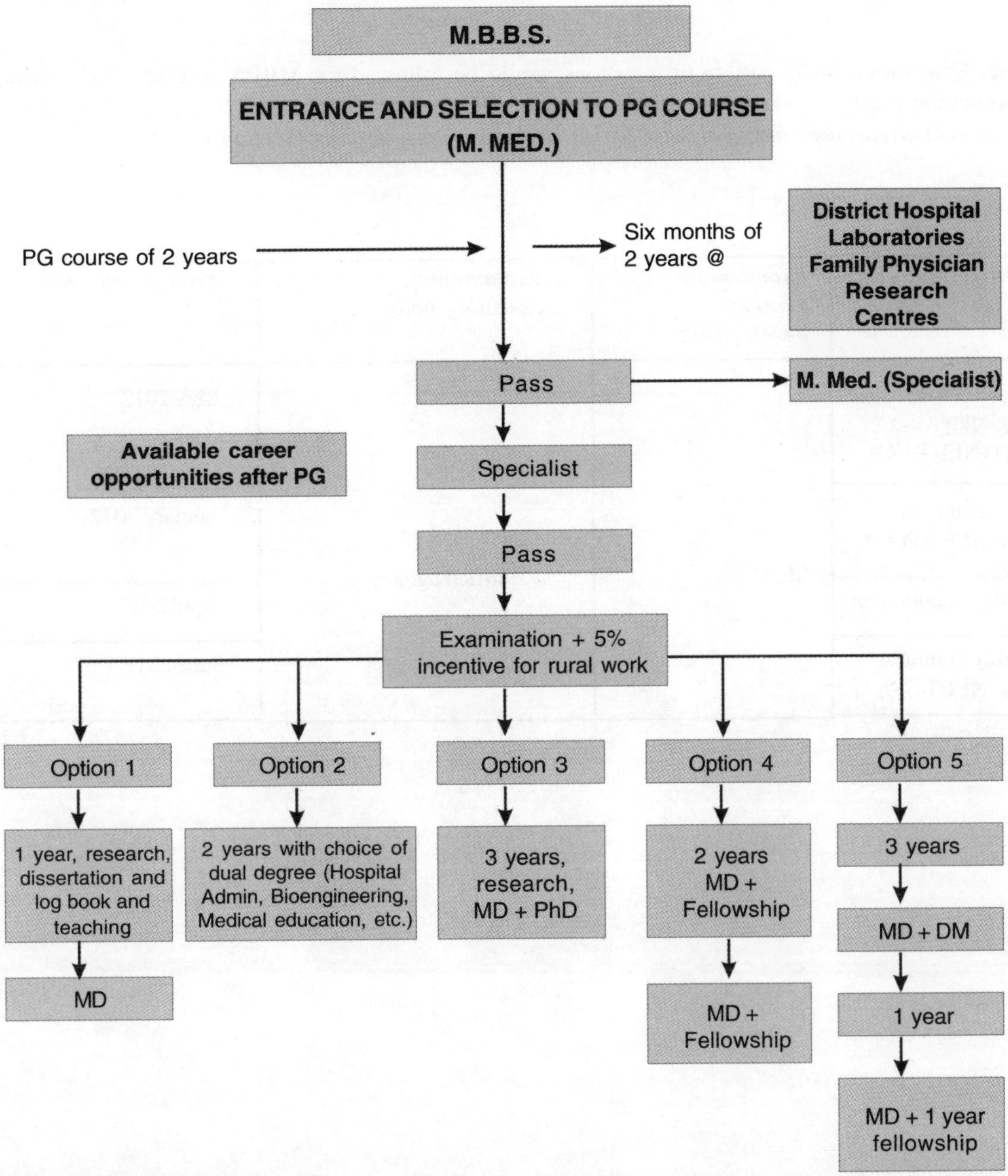

DURATION OF VARIOUS PG COURSES

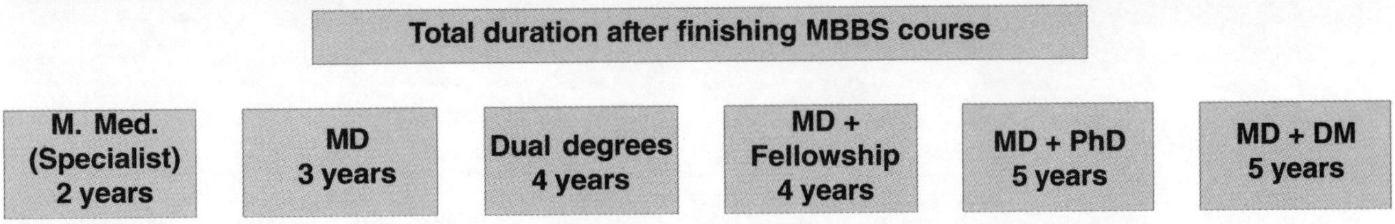

Type of Paper/Questions: MCQ pattern of questions would be followed for MBBS entrance. The PG and DM/MCh entrance examination papers *would have multiple types of MCQs, namely single response (Section A-60%), multiple T/F, images, assertion/reasoning questions and patient management questions (Section B-40%).*

Examination	*Examination content development*	*Examination executing body*	*First examination*
Undergraduate (UG) National Eligibility-cum-Entrance Test (NEET-UG)	MCI	Identified agency	May 2012
Postgraduate common entrance test–NEET-PG			January 2012
Licentiate IMG examination			April 2013
Superspeciality common entrance test–NEET-SS			June 2012

CONTENTS

(All MCQs asked in various exams are answered on the basis of the text of the book which is sourced from standard Dermatology, Leprosy and STD books and national and international guidelines).

Mock Test Based on Proposed CET 2012 (MCI)

(All images are from the Comprehensive Textbook of Dermatology*–Garg, Sardana, Published by Peepee Publishers and Distributors (P) Ltd. The *only* book with 360° coverage of topics for dermatology MCQ with the maximum and most comprehensive source of images)

1. **The cell marked in Fig. 1 is:**
   A. S corneum B. S granulosum
   C. S basale D. S malphigian

2. **Assertion: In psoriasis the cell proliferation is fast. Reasoning: This leads to increase in S granulosum layer.**
   A. The assertion is right reasoning is wrong
   B. Both the statements are wrong
   C. The assertion is wrong reasoning is right
   D. Both are wrong

3. **The marked (dark line) in Fig. 2 refers to:**
   A. Kertain B. Desmosome
   C. Lamina densa D. Acantholysis

4. **With regard to acantholysis please mark (T/F) of the following statements:**
   A. It is same as dyskeratosis
   B. It is seen in herpes infection
   C. Primary acantholysis is seen in pemphigus
   D. Damage to desmosomes is seen in Darier's disease

5. **Which is the type of granuloma described in Fig. 3?**
   A. Naked granuloma
   B. Tuberculoid granuloma
   C. Sarcoidal granuloma
   D. Suppurative granuloma

6. **A patient comes with itchy nodules on the scrotum Fig. 4. What is the most likely diagnosis?**
   A. Prurigo
   B. Lichen simplex chronicus
   C. Darier's disease
   D. Clean man scabies

7. **Assertion: Sulfur is the DOC for Scabies in pregnancy. Reasoning: Sulfur is the safest but not the most effective drug in scabies.**
   A. The assertion is right reasoning is right
   B. Both the statements are wrong
   C. The assertion is wrong reasoning is right
   D. Both the statements are right

8. **Please identify the likely diagnosis of a case presenting to the STD in Fig. 5:**
   A. Syphilis B. Herpes
   C. Chancroid D. Aphthous ulcers

* Approved by MCI for Diploma Skin Degree.

9. **The cell is Fig. 6 is:**
   A. Acantholytic cell B. Tzanck cell
   C. Clue cell D. Dyskeratotic cell

10. **Which of the following is seen in early congenital syphilis (T/F):**
    A. Parrots pseudoparalysis
    B. Clutton joints
    C. Parrots lines
    D. Hutchinson teeth

11. **Identify the lesion in the picture Fig. 7**
    A. Purpura B. Vasculitis
    C. Target lesion D. Macule

12. **A patient comes with annular plaque with central scarring and peripheral pigmentation on the face with a positive ss DNA (Fig. 8). What is the diagnosis?**
    A. Lupus vulgaris B. SLE
    C. DM D. DLE

13. **Assertion: Atopic dermatitis is characterised by itching. Reasoning: AD has an onset after 3 months.**
    A. Assertion is right and reasoning is right
    B. Assertion is wrong and reasoning is right
    C. Assertion is right and reasoning is wrong
    D. Both assertion and reasoning are wrong

14. **A male patient presents with flaccid bulla and a biopsy is sent for evaluation (Fig. 9). What is the finding?**
    A. Subepidermal blister
    B. Suprabasal acantholysis
    C. Subcorenal blister
    D. Lichenoid infiltrate

15. **An elderly male has urticaria with superimposed bulla (Fig. 10). The DIF reveals a linear IgG. What is the diagnosis?**
    A. Pemphigus B. DH
    C. Linear Ig A disease D. BP

16. **Which of the following is T (True) or F (False) regarding DH?**
    A. Wheat aggravates DH
    B. Dapsone is the drug of choice
    C. Glutein free diet is curative
    D. The antigen is TG 2

17. Assertion: DIF in a case of epidermolysis bullosa is negative.
Reasoning: It is a mechanobullous disorders.
A. Assertion is right and reasoning is right
B. Assertion is wrong and reasoning is right
C. Assertion is right and reasoning is wrong
D. Both assertion and reasoning are wrong

18. Please mark T (True) or F (False):
A. Antigen of pemphigus vulgaris is desmoglein 1
B. Antigen of bullous pemphigoid is desmoglein 3
C. The antigen of BP is unknown
D. Pemphigus vegetans is a variant of P foliaceus

19. Which test is being demonstrated in Fig. 11?
A. Diascopy B. Grattage test
C. Dariers sign D. Dermatographism

20. In the test in Fig. 11 what is the final diagnois?
A. Psoriasis B. Lichen planus
C. Urticaria D. Purpura

21. What is the best therapy for the patient in Fig. 12?
A. PUVA B. NBUVB
C. Tar D. Steroids

22. The patient in Fig. 13 has an asymptomatic papulo-squamous rash which is arranged along the rib cage. The biopsy revealed a psoriasiform pathology. What is the most likely diagnosis?
A. PRP B. Drug rash
C. Secondary syphilis D. P rosea

23. What does the classic pattern shown in Fig. 14 refer to?
A. Erosions B. Leukoplakia
C. Thrush D. Wickham's striae

24. The patient in Fig. 15 came with bone defects and multiple tumours and large brownish spots on the back. What is the diagnosis?
A. Lichen planus B. Leprosy
C. Psoriasis D. NF

25. A case with epiloia comes with the findings as seen in Fig. 16. What is it ?
A. Adenoma sebaceum B. CALM
C. Crowe's signs D. Koenen tumours

26. The patient in Fig. 17 has loss of hair with absent hair follicles and the biopsy revealed fibrosis. The case was labelled as a idiopathic alopecia. What is the diagnosis?
A. Lichen planus B. Alopecia areata
C. Kerion D. Pseudopelade

27. What is the pathognomic change that is represented in Fig. 18?
A. Pterygium B. Koilonychia
C. Pittings D. Oil drop sign

28. The patient in Fig. 19 had yellowish concretions in the axilla the KOH was negative. The diagnosis is:
A. Psoriasis B. Piedra
C. Trichomycosis axillaris D. Chromhidrosis

29. A patient comes with white scaly plaques on the trunk the KOH is given in Fig. 20. Please mark the statements that are T/F:
A. The slide shows pseudophyphae
B. The slide shows hyphae
C. It's a case of psoriasis
D. Both hyphae and spores are seen

30. A farmer comes with a painless, firm papule or papulopustule which forms a plaque with a warty look (Fig. 21). The diagnosis is:
A. Psoriasis B. Leprosy
C. ENL D. TBVC

31. A patient comes with a plaque (Fig. 22) which is anesthetic, lepromin + and slit smear negative. The diagnosis is:
A. IL B. TT
C. BT D. BB

32. The marked phenomenon in Fig. 23 refers to:
A. Reaction B. ENL
C. Neuritis D. Satellite phenomenon

33. The patient in Fig. 23 is slit smear positive, what drugs will you give?
A. ROM therapy B. MB MDT
C. PB MDT D. Wait and Watch

34. Assertion: The drug of choice for sever ENL is thalidomide.
Reasoning: Thalidomide inhibits TNF α:
A. Assertion is right and reasoning is right
B. Assertion is wrong and reasoning is right
C. 0Assertion is right and reasoning is wrong
D. Both assertion and reasoning is wrong

Answers :

1. B	2. A	3. B	4. A–F, B–T, C–T, D–F
5. A	6. D	7. A	8. C
9. B	10. A–T, B–F, C–F, D–F	11. C	12. D
13. C	14. B	15. D	16. A–T, B–T, C–F, D–T
17. A	18. A–F, B–F, C–F, D–F	19. A	20. D
21. B	22. D	23. D	24. D
25. D	26. D	27. D	28. C
29. A–F, B–F, C–F, D–T	30. D	31. B	32. D
33. B	34. A		

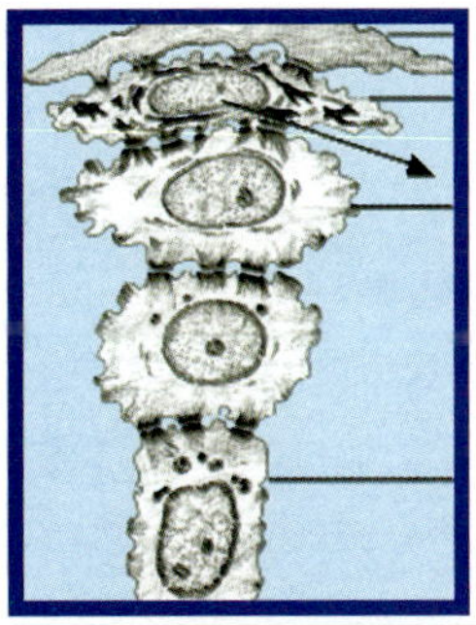

Fig. 1

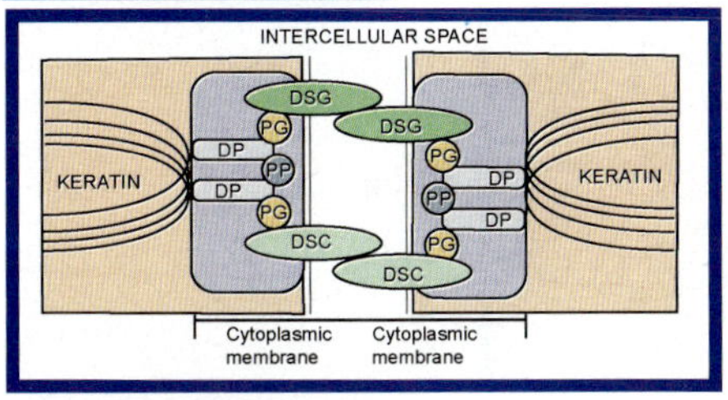

Fig. 2

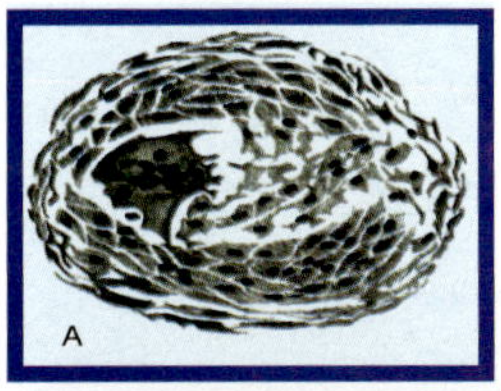

Fig. 3

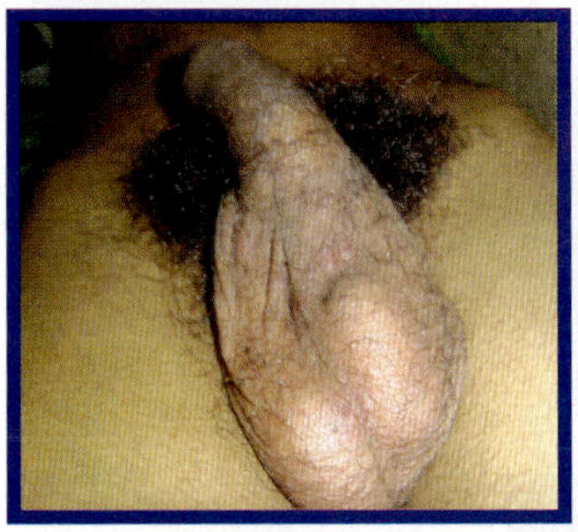

Fig. 4

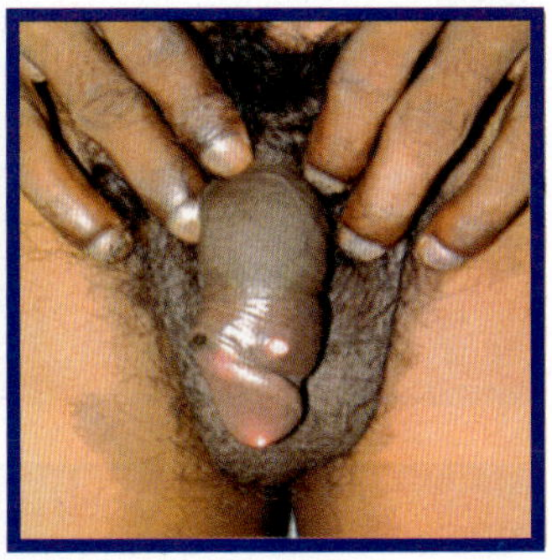

Fig. 5

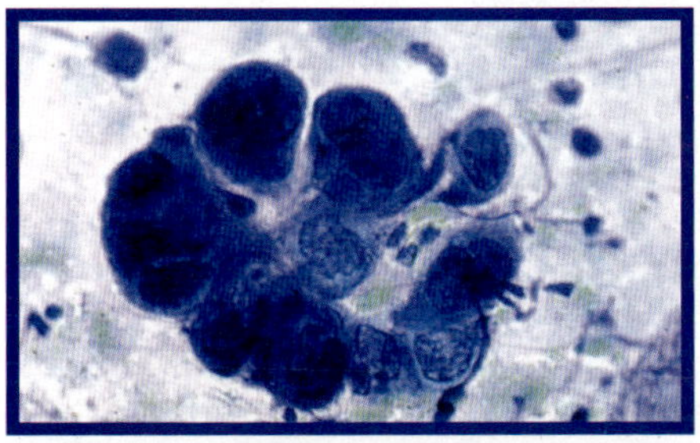

Fig. 6

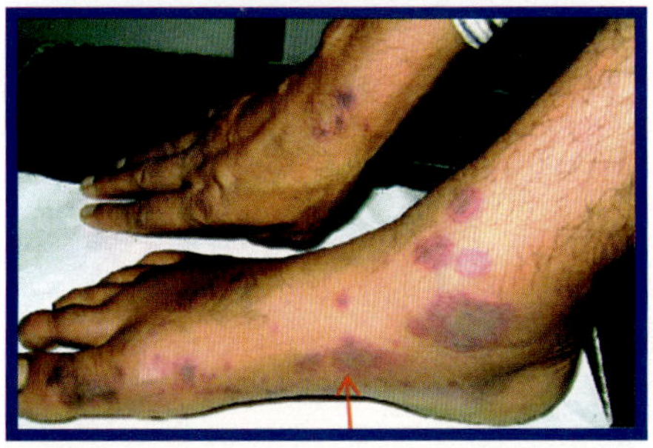

Fig. 7

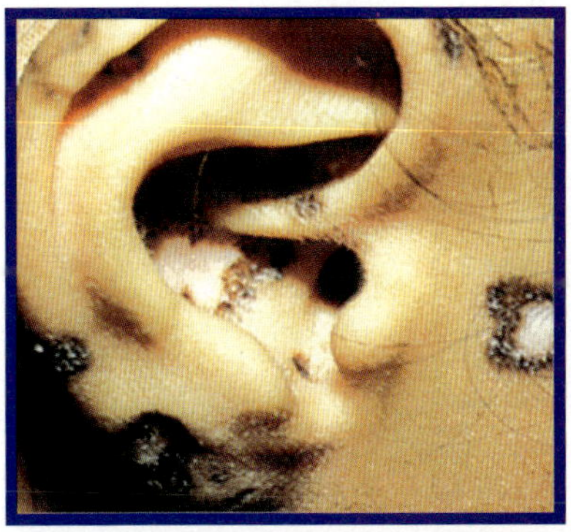

Fig. 8

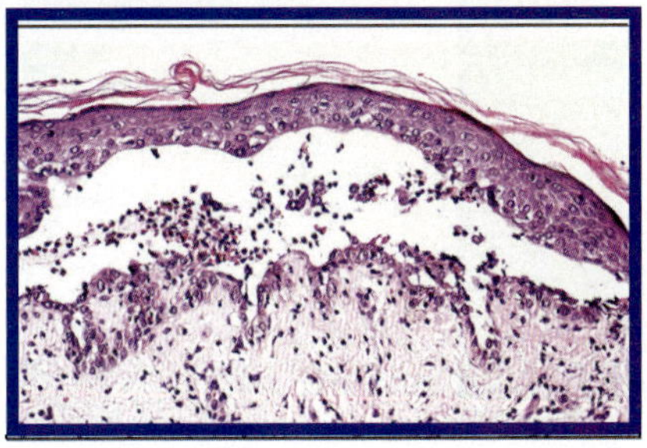

Fig. 9

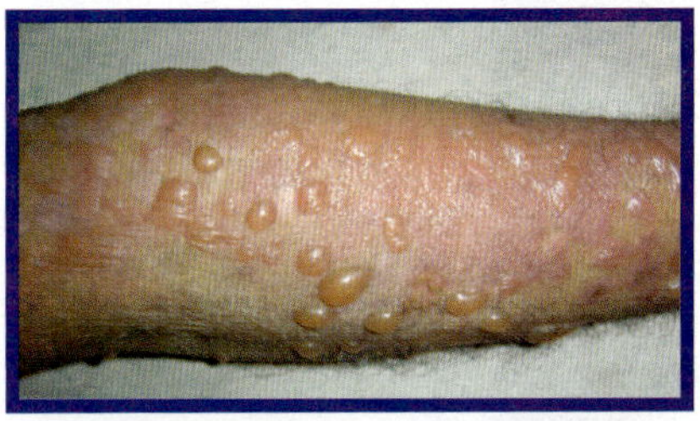

Fig. 10

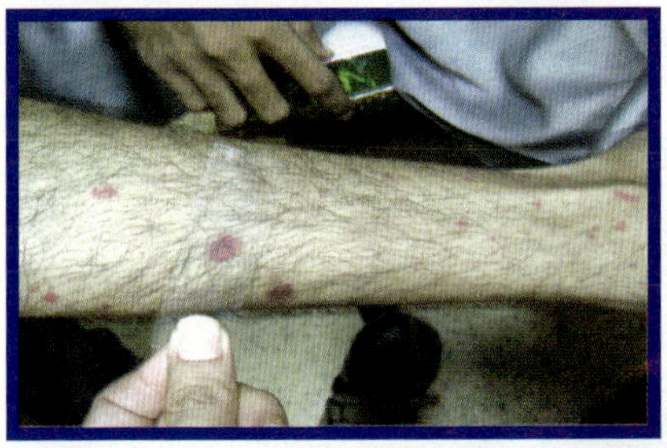

Fig. 11

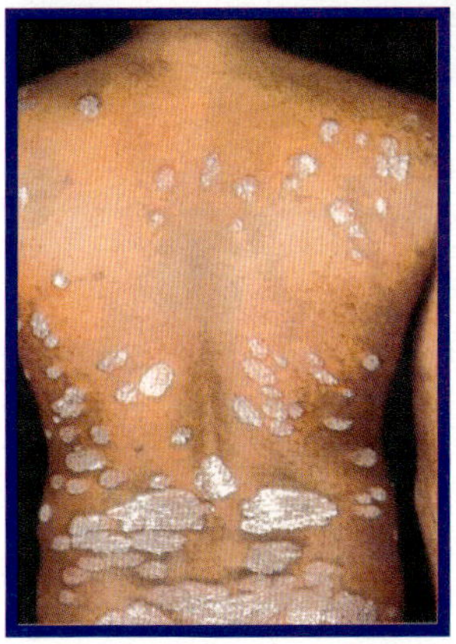

Fig. 12

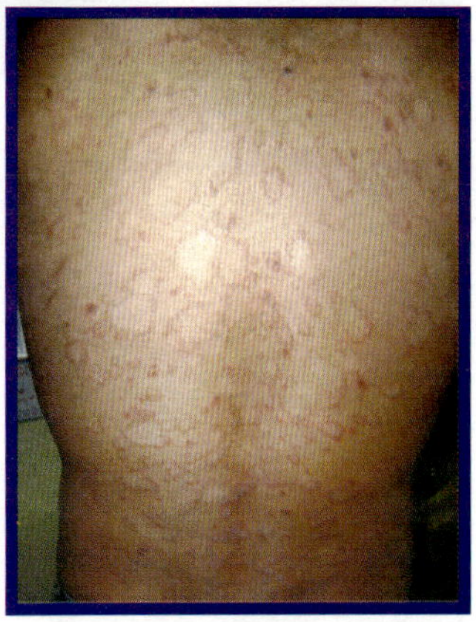

Fig. 13

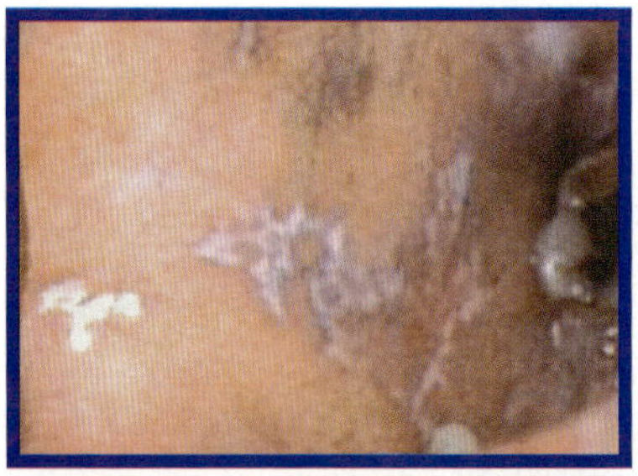
Fig. 14

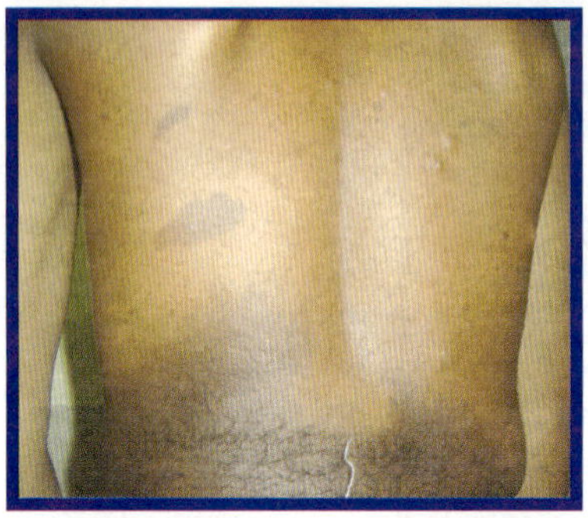
Fig. 15

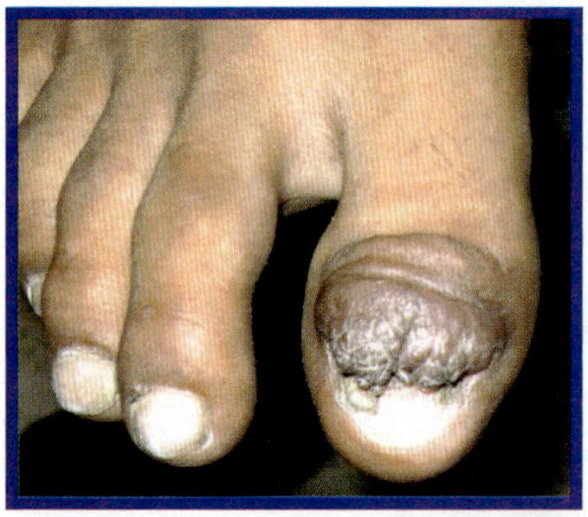
Fig. 16

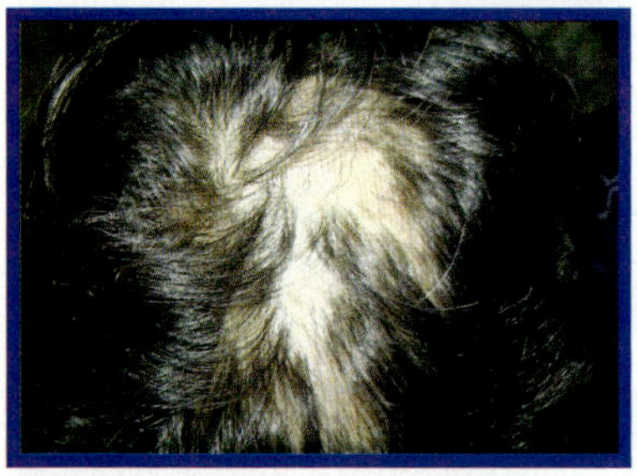
Fig. 17

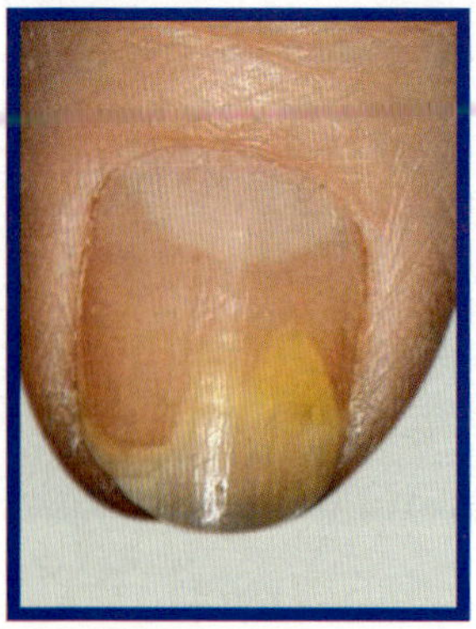
Fig. 18

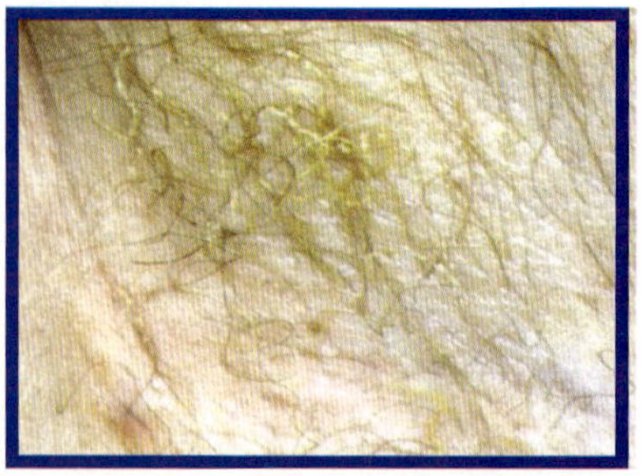
Fig. 19

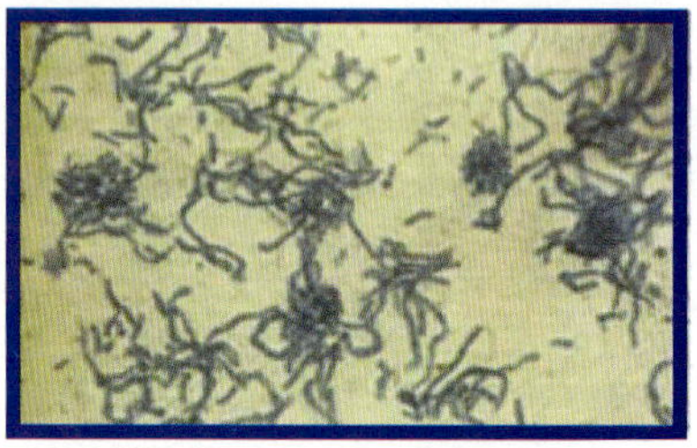
Fig. 20

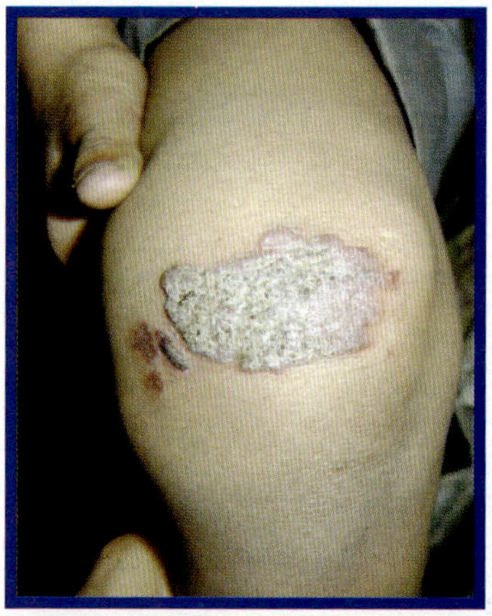
Fig. 21

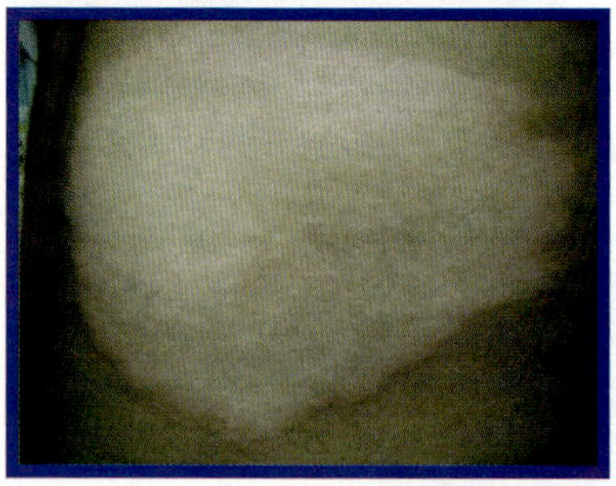
Fig. 22

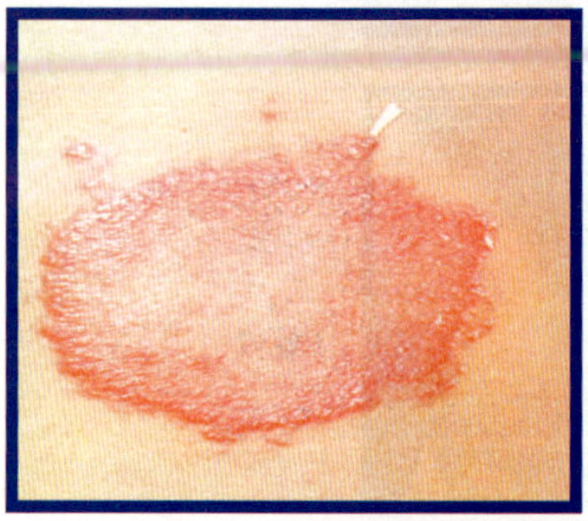
Fig. 23

Part I

Exam MCQs asked from
***MCQs in Dermatology*, First edition (2009-11)**
by *Sardana* and *Garg*

JIPMER (60%), AIIMS (50%)
AIPG (50%), Delhi PG (75%), UPSC (72%)

Exam MCQs asked from *MCQs in Dermatology,* First edition (2009-11) by *Sardana* and *Garg*

JIPMER (60%), AIIMS (50%)
AIPG (50%), Delhi PG (75%), UPSC (72%)

The MCQs ticked are those from the 1st edn. of the MCQs book. The *Comprehensive Textbook of Dermatology : Garg VK., Sardana K., Peepee Publishers* has the unique distinction of being the ONLY BOOK based on Standard Books and 100% of MCQs of exams in last 2 years are from the Book !

AIIMS (MAY 2011)

√1. In congenital dystrophic variety of epidermolysis bullosa, mutation is seen in the gene conding for:

A. Laminin 4
B. Collagen type 7
C. Alpha 6 integrin
D. Keratin 14

2. Histopathological features of fat necrosis in a newborn closely resembles:

A. Steroid induced lipid necrosis
B. Lupoid necrosis
C. Erythema induratum
D. Lipodermatosclerosis

√3. True about incontinenta pigmenti include the following *except*:

A. X-linked dominant
B. Primary skin abnormality
C. Avascularity of peripheral retina
D. Ocular involvement is seen in almost 100% cases and is typically unilateral

√4. Which is false about acrodermatitis enteropathica?

A. Triad of diarrhoea, dementia and dermatitis
B. Low serum zinc levels
C. Symptoms improve with zinc supplementation
D. Autosomal recessive

√5. Child presents with linear verrucous plaques on the trunk with vacuolization of keratinocytes in S. Spinosum and S. Granulosum. Diagnosis is:

A. Incontinenta pigmenti
B. Delayed hypersensitivity reaction
C. Verrucous epidermal nevus
D. Linear darier's disease

6. Girl 2 years coming with bosselated erythematous lesion on right cheek, what is treatment of choice?

A. Pulse dye laser
B. Nd Yag
C. CO_2 / Yetterium
D. Switched ruby laser

7. Patient with fine reticular rashes with palmar pigmentation, what is the diagnosis?

A. Downling Dego syndrome
B. Rothmind Thompson syndrome
C. Cockyane syndrome
D. Bloom syndrome

√8. A pregnant gets chickenpox 3 days before delivery of the baby. What is the baby's prognosis?

A. No risk to mother or child
B. Intrapartum antiviral therapy required
C. Fetopathic effects seen
D. At risk of fetal varicella syndrome

Answers :

1. (B)	**2. (A)**	**3. (D)**	**4. (A)**	**5. (C)**
6. (A)	**7. (A)**	**8. (B)**		

AIIMS (NOVEMBER–DECEMBER 2010)

√1. A teen age girl with moderate acne also complaining of irregular menses. Drug of choice will be:

A. Oral isotretinoin
B. Oral acitretin
C. Oral minocycline
D. Cyproterone acetate

2. Malignant pustule is seen in:

A. Anthrax
B. Basal cell carcinoma
C. Squamous cell carcinoma
D. Rapidly spreading rodent ulcer

3. Chemical peeling is not done by all *except*:

A. Trichloroacetic acid
B. Phosphoric acid
C. Carboxylic acid
D. Kojic acid

√4. Farmer with single verrucous plaque on leg. Which of the following could be the lesion?

A. Verruca vulgaris
B. Tuberculosis verrucosa cutis
C. Mycetoma
D. Lichen planus hypertrophicus

√5. 25 years old labourer 3 years back presented with penile ulcer not treated. Later he presented with neurological symptoms for which he got treated. Test to monitor response to treatment is:

A. VDRL B. FTA ABS
C. TPI D. RPR

Answers :

1. (A) 2. (A) 3. (A) 4. (B) 5. (A)

AIIMS (MAY 2010)

√1. Which of the following is not true about lepromin test?

A. It is diagnostic
B. It is negative in infants less than 6 months
C. It is used to classify leprosy
D. BCG vaccination may convert negative to positive

√2. Leprosy affects all of the following *except*:

A. Uterus
B. Eyes
C. Ovaries
D. Nerves

3. What is the most specific test for syphilis?

A. VDRL
B. RPR
C. FTA-Abs
D. Kahn's test

√4. A middle aged man presented with ulcerative granuloma on glans. Wright Giemsa stain showed 1-2 rounded structures in macrophage vacuoles. What is the etiologic agent?

A. Chlamydia trachomatis
B. Neisseria gonorrheae
C. Calymmatobacterium granulomatis
D. Staphylococcus aureus

5. Thalidomide is used in all of the following *except*:

A. HIV associated peripheral neuropathy
B. HIV associated aphthous (mouth) ulcers
C. Behcet syndrome
D. Erythema nodosum leprosum

6. A 25-year-old male had arthritis in right ankle and multiple erythematous nodules on the shin. He had fever and malaise for 2 weeks. What is the likely diagnosis?

A. Erythema nodosum
B. Hensen's disease
C. Weber Christian disease
D. Urticarial vasculitis

7. Strawberry gingiva is seen in which of the following?

A. Wegener's granulomatosis
B. Monocytic leukemia
C. Phenytoin gum hypertrophy
D. Klippel Trenauney syndrome

8. Which of the following is not a primary cutaneous disorder?

A. Psoriasis
B. Lichen planus
C. Reiter disease
D. Icthyosis

√9. A child presents with recurrent episodes of lip edema and laryngeal edema and abdominal pain associated with stress. Levels of which of the following are reduced?

A. C1 esterase inhibitor B. C5a
C. C3 D. C9

Answers :

1. (A)	2. (C)	3. (C)	4. (C)	5. (A)
6. (A)	7. (A)	8. (C)	9. (A)	

AIIMS NOVEMBER 2009

√1. Defective DNA repair is seen in:

A. Xeroderma pigmentosum
B. Albinism
C. Vitiligo
D. N achromicus

√2. Treatment of choice in genital wart in pregnancy:

A. Salicylic acid with lactic acid solution
B. Podophyllotoxin
C. Imiqimod
D. Cryotherapy

√3. Recurrent plaques on glans which heal with residual hyperpigmentation (Skin):

A. Apthous ulcer
B. Fixed drug eruption
C. Herpes gestationalis
D. Chlamydial inf.

√4. 10 years old boy with scalp boggy swelling with multiple sinuses, easy pluckable hair, lymph nodes enlarged in occipital region, diagnosis is made by:

A. Biopsy B. Culture
C. KOH D. Wood's lamp

√5. Which of the following not seen in dermatomyositis?

A. Gottron's papules
B. Periungual telangiectasia
C. Salmon rash
D. Mechanics hand

6. Necrotizing lymphadenitis is:

A. Kimura's disease B. Kikuchi's disease
C. Castleman's disease D. Sturge-Weber syndrome

√7. Which of the following is not true about Neisseria gonorrheae?

A. Most common manifestation in men is urethritis
B. Uniformly sensitive to penicillin
C. Exclusive human pathogen
D. Some strains may cause disseminated disease

√8. Not a common cause of vasculitis in adults:

A. Giant cell arteritis B. PAN
C. Kawasaki disease D. HSP

√9. HPV vaccine is:

A. Monovalent B. Bivalent
C. Trivalent D. Quadrivalent

Answers :

1. (A)	2. (D)	3. (B)	4. (B)	5. (C)
6. (B)	7. (B)	8. (D)	9. (D)	

ALL INDIA PG (JANUARY 2011)

1. Lines of blaschko are:

A. Lymphatics
B. Blood vessel
C. Nerves
D. Lines of development

√2. Clue cells are seen in:

A. Bacterial vaginosis
B. Vaginal candidiasis
C. Chlamydial vaginosis
D. Trichomoniasis

3. Pregnant mother at 35 weeks of gestation. What drug can you not give her for treatment of SLE?

A. Prednisolone B. Methotrexate
C. Sulfasalazine D. Hydroxychloroquine

√4. A young male presented with history of fever and a nodule in the leg. Histopathology of the nodule revealed foamy histiocytes and neutrophilic infiltrate in the dermis. Most probable diagnosis is:

A. Sweet's syndrome
B. Rosai Dorfman disease
C. Erythema nodosum leprosum
D. E indurativum

√5. **Cicatricing alopecia with perifollicular violaceous hue is commonly associated with all *except*:**

A. Nail dystrophy
B. Whitish lesion in the buccal mucosa
C. Arthritis
D. Discoid plaques in the face

6. **Pseudoisomorphic phenomenon seen in:**

A. Psoriasis B. Lichen planus
C. Vitiligo D. Plane warts

Answers :
1. (D) 2. (A) 3. (B) 4. (C) 5. (C) 6. (A)

AIPG 2010

1. **Steroid most potent as:**

A. Cream B. Ointment
C. Lotion D. Gel

√2. **Treatment of erythematous rash in pregnant female:**

A. Corticosteroid B. Isotretinoin
C. MTX D. Psoralen with PUVA

√3. **Child with history of infantile spasm, hypopigmented macule on back, delayed milestone:**

A. Tuberous sclerosis B. NF
C. Sturge-Weber D. N anemicus

√4. **While lacy lesion in oral cavity with extension of proximal nail fold onto the nail plate:**

A. Lichen planus B. FDE
C. SLE D. Dermatophytosis

5. **A female with pimples, treatment resulting in pigmentation, which drug is given?**

A. Tetracycline B. Erythromycin
C. Minocycline D. Doxycycline

Answers :
1. (B) 2. (A) 3. (A) 4. (A) 5. (C)

DELHI PG 2011

1. **Grenz zone is found in all, *except:***

A. Lepromatous leprosy B. Granuloma faciale
C. Granuloma annulare D. Lymphocytoma

2. **All of the following are dermatological adverse effects of topically administered steroids, *except:***

A. Intertrigo B. Skin atrophy
C. Superinfection D. Telangiectasia

3. **A skin test can show hypersensitivity reactions of all the following types *except:***

A. Type I B. Type II
C. Type III D. Type IV

4. **Which of the following parameters is not monitored in a patient on methotrexate therapy?**

A. Liver function tests B. Lung function test
C. Eye examination D. Hemogram

√5. **Whiff test is used to detect:**

A. Trichomoniasis B. Candidal cervicitis
C. Bacterial vaginosis D. Gonococcal cervicitis

√6. **Patch test is read after:**

A. 2 hours B. 2 days
C. 2 weeks D. 2 months

√7. **School of fish appearance is shown by:**

A. Hemqophilus ducreyi B. Gonococcus
C. Chalmydia D. Donovania granulomatis

√8. **A person presenting 5 days after contact with a commercial sexual partner with complaints of multiple penile ulcers, suppurative inguinal lymph node is suffering from:**

A. Secondary syphilis B. Chancroid
C. LGV D. Primary herpes

√9. **A 27 years old male had burning micturition and urethral discharge. After 4 weeks he developed joint pain involving both the knees and ankles, redness of the eye and skin lesions. The most probable clinical diagnosis is:**

A. Psoriasis vulgaris B. Reiter's syndrome
C. Behcet's syndrome D. Sarcoidosis

√10. A 45 years old farmer has itchy erythematous papular lesions on face, neck, "V" area of chest, dorsum of hands and forearms for 3 years. The lesions are more severer in summers and improve by 75% in winters. The most appropriate test to diagnose the condition would be:
A. Skin biopsy
B. Estimation of IgE levels in blood
C. Patch test
D. Intradermal prick test

√11. A 40 years old male reported with recurrent episodes of oral ulcers, large areas of denuded skin and flaccid vesiculobullous eruptions. Which is the most important bed side investigation helpful in establishing the diagnosis?
A. Gram staining of the blister fluid
B. Culture and sensitivity
C. Skin biopsy and immunofluorescence
D. Tzanck smear from the floor of bulla

√12. A patient had severe irregular hyperpigmented macules on the trunk and multiple small hyperpigmented macules in the axillae and groins since early childhood. There were no other skin lesions. Which is the most likely investigation to support the diagnosis?
A. Slit-lamp examination of eye
B. Measurement of intraocular tension
C. Examination of fundus
D. Retinal artery angiography

13. All the following are causes of "lupus" *except:*
A. Hydralazine B. Clofibrate
C. Penicillamine D. Chlorpromazine

√14. Degeneration of basal cells occurs in:
A. Lichen planus B. Pemphigus
C. Psoriasis D. Pemphigoid

15. Most common side effect of dapsone:
A. Hemlyticanemia
B. Thrombocytopenia
C. Cyanosis
D. Bone marrow depression

16. 8 years old male child with recurrent scaly hypo -pigmented macules on the face. Diagnosis is:
A. Pityriasis alba
B. Leprosy
C. Tinea versicolor
D. Pityriasis roseace

√17. PUVA therapy is used in:
A. Psoriasis
B. Lichen planus
C. Freckles
D. Melasma

Answers :

1. (C)	2. (A)	3. (B)	4. (C)	5. (C)
6. (B)	7. (A)	8. (B)	9. (B)	10. (C)
11. (D)	12. (A)	13. (B)	14. (A)	15. (A)
16. (A)	17. (A)			

DELHI PG (FEBRUARY 2010)

√1. A pinkish red fluorescence of urine in Wood's lamp is seen in:
A. Lead poisoning B. PCT
C. Erythromelalgia D. Acrocyanosis

√2. Griseofulvin is not used in one of the following:
A. T capitis B. T cruris
C. T versicolor D. T pedis

3. Causative organism of molluscum contagiosum is:
A. Papova virus B. Pox virus
C. Parvo virus D. Orthomyxo virus

√4. The most characteristic finding in lichen planus is:
A. Civatte bodies
B. Basal cell degeneration
C. Thinning of nail plate
D. Violaceous lesions

√5. Which of the following caused alopecia without scarring?
A. LE B. Herpes zoster
C. Alopecia areata D. Lichen planus

6. Erythema multiforme is associated with:
A. Herpes zoster B. Herpes simplex
C. Molluscum D. HPV

√7. A 25-year-old male had pigmented macules on the palm, sole and oral mucosa with pain abdomen the diagnosis is:

A. Albright syndrome
B. Cushing's syndrome
C. Peutz-Jeghers syndrome
D. Incontinentia pigmentii

√8. **Treatment of choice in solar keratosis:**
A. Methotrexate
B. Topical 5 FU
C. Topical mechlorethamine
D. Steroids

9. **All of the following hematological disorders cause pruritus *except*:**
A. PCV
B. Hemolytic anemia
C. Multiple myeloma
D. NHL

√10. **Darier's sign is seen in:**
A. Xenoderma pigmentosa
B. Urticaria pigmentosa
C. Herpes zoster
D. Glucagonoma

√11. **Erythema marginatum is seen in:**
A. Drug reactions
B. Typhus fever
C. Enteric fever
D. Rheumatic fever

√12. **Nail involvement is not seen in:**
A. Dermatophytosis
B. Lichen planus
C. DLE
D. Psoriasis

Answers :

1. (B) 2. (C) 3. (B) 4. (C) 5. (C)
6. (B) 7. (C) 8. (B) 9. (B) 10. (B)
11. (D) 12. (C)

UPSC 2010

√1. **Acrodermatitis enetropthaica is associated with the deficiency of:**
A. Copper
B. Cobalt
C. Chromium
D. ZN

√2. **A 4-year-old child is admitted with fever, conjunctivitis, rashes, cervical LN, heptomegaly and desquamation of fingers and toes. Echo shows coronoary artery aneurysm, the likely diagnosis is:**
A. Measles
B. German measles
C. Progeria
D. Kawasaki disease

3. **The clinical features of congenital syphilis in neonatal period include the following *except*:**
A. Interstitial keratitis
B. Choroiditis
C. Meningitis
D. Osteochondritis

√4. **In which stage of syphilis are the lesions of condyloma lata present?**
A. Primary
B. Secondary
C. Tertiary
D. Congenital

√5. **A cystic boggy swelling over the scalp in a child with partial or complete alopecia:**
A. Folliculitis decalvans
B. Hematoma
C. Kerion
D. Congenital syphilis

√6. **The earliest sensation to be lost in leprosy is:**
A. Thermal
B. Tactile
C. Pain
D. Vibration

7. **What is the causative virus for common wart?**
A. HPV
B. CMV
C. HIV
D. HSV

√8. **Wood's light is helpful in recognition of ash leaf spots in patients with:**
A. Atopic dermatitis
B. Lichen planus
C. Nummular eczema
D. Tuberous sclerosis

9. **An AIDS patient of TB lymphadenitis is on HAART and has an increase in size of lymph nodes with a doubling of CD 4 count, the diagnosis is:**
A. Multidrug persistent TB
B. Drug defaulter for ATT
C. IRIS
D. Poor compliance

√10. **A man present with recurrent episodes old pruritic vesicles symmetrically distributed on the trunk. DIF shows IgA granular pattern on the BMZ. Which of the following is associated with it?**
A. Celiac sprue
B. Lactase deficiency
C. Whipple's disease
D. Ulcerative colitis

√11. **Painless genital ulcer are seen in:**
A. Granuloma inguinale
B. Chancroid
C. LGV
D. HSV

Answers :

1. (D) 2. (D) 3. (A) 4. (B) 5. (C)
6. (A) 7. (D) 8. (C) 9. (C) 10. (A)
11. (A)

JIPMER (FEBRUARY 2010)

√1. **Xeroderma pigmentosa the defect is in:**
A. Mismath repair
B. Nucleotide excison repair
C. Ds DNA break repair
D. Chromosomal defect

2. **Vitiligo is associated with:**
A. DM
B. Hypothyroidism
C. DI
D. Nail disorders

√3. **Fish net appearance is seen in:**
A. P vulgaris
B. Bullous pemphigoid
C. DH
D. CP

4. **Ivermectin is used in all *except*:**
A. Scabies
B. Onchocercosis
C. Filaria
D. Malaria

5. **Toxic shock syndrome is caused because of:**
A. Superantigen
B. PVL
C. Hemolytic toxin
D. Type 1 response

√6. **Beefy red ulcer with foul smelling discharge is seen in:**
A. Chancroid
B. Donovaniosis
C. Syphilis
D. Herpers

7. **Leukonychia is seen in:**
A. Lead poisoning
B. Zn deficiency
C. Hypoalbuminemia
D. Iron deficiency anemia

√8. **Oral PUVA is used in all *except*:**
A. Vitiligo
B. MF
C. Melasma
D. Psoriasis

9. **Brownish staining of the teeth in a child fluoresces in UV light is because of:**
A. Porphyria
B. Tetracycline
C. Dentogenic defect
D. Gunther's disease

√10. **Oral hairy Leukoplakia is caused by:**
A. EBV
B. Candida
C. CMV
D. HSV

√11. **All are seen in dermatomyositis *except:***
A. Gottron's papules
B. Shwal sign
C. Calcinosis cutis
D. Heliotrope sign

12. **HPV vaccine is composed of the following HPV:**
A. 11,6,18,16
B. 11,16,31,35
C. 11,6,35,16
D. 38,31,16,18

Answers :

1. (B)	**2. (A)**	**3. (A)**	**4. (D)**	**5. (A)**
6. (B)	**7. (C)**	**8. (C)**	**9. (B)**	**10. (A)**
11. (C)	**12. (A)**			

Answers of MCQs asked in exams of 2009-2011

We will be giving answers of the difficult or controversial Q. only. The answers are from STANDARD TEXTBOOKS and *every single Q. asked in the last 2 years* has detailed explanations in the *Comprehensive Textbook of Dermatology (Garg, Sardana) Peepee Publishers*. This is because this book was written primarily with MCQs in mind.

No other book of Dermatology for Undergraduate students has correct answers as they are either incomplete, repetitive or were never written for MCQs.

AIPG JANUARY 2011

Q. 3. Pregnant mother at 35 weeks of gestation. What drug can you not give her for treatment of SLE?

Pregnancy in Patients with SLE

- Aside from the fetal risks associated with anti-Ro autoimmunity, pregnant patients with SLE present special concerns. Pregnancy may proceed without complication in patients with inactive SLE, though pregnancy may also induce a flare of the disease.
- The main risk factors that may lead to complications and affect the course and outcome of pregnancy are *active disease, hypertension and nephritis*. SLE can be associated with increased hypertensive complications, preterm birth, low birth weight and stillbirth, and the degree of risk correlates with the severity of maternal disease. Recurrent pregnancy loss is particularly associated with antiphospholipid antibody syndrome. In addition, the management of active SLE is hampered by the possible adverse effects of immunosuppressive medications on the fetus.
- It is recommended that pregnant women with SLE should undergo frequent ultrasonographic examinations and the fetal heart rate should be monitored during the second and third trimesters.

Antimalarials (AMs)

Antimalarial drugs (AMs), mainly chloroquine (CQ) and hydroxychloroquine (HCQ), are primarily indicated in SLE patients with non-life-threatening organ involvement, especially for arthritis and skin rashes. Hydroxychloroquine was identified as an adjuvant treatment for achieving remission in lupus nephritis in two retrospective studies. Apart from the prevention of flares of the disease, multiple, large, prospective studies have shown that AMs reduce the extent of irreversible organ damage and confer an overall survival benefit to patients with SLE with a more than 50% reduction in mortality rate. Other reported beneficial effects of AMs in SLE include a reduction in severity of atherosclerosis, antithrombotic effect, improvement in bone mineral density and a reduction in the risk of cancer The adverse effects of AMs when used in SLE patients and other rheumatological indications are mild, and are mainly gastrointestinal and cutaneous. The only study comparing the toxicity of CQ and HCQ, found a higher frequency of adverse effects with CQ (28.4% vs 14.7%). An analysis obtained from various studies has shown that treatment with CQ for a mean duration of 10 years resulted in retinal toxicity in 16/647 i.e. 2.5% patients, compared with only 2/2043 i.e. 0.1% patients developing it during treatment with HCQ for a similar duration. Antimalarials are ***safe for the fetus when given to the pregnant mother, with no cases of fetal malformations have been reported beyond those that were normally expected.***

Given their efficacy and safety profile, AMs, preferably HCQ, should be prescribed universally to all patients with SLE, starting as soon as the diagnosis has been made and maintained for an indefinite period. Antimalarial therapy should not be stopped even if the patient develops a more serious organic lupus involvement, and irrespective of the addition of aggressive immunosuppressive treatments. Regular ophthalmological assessments are important for the early detection of retinal and other ocular adverse effects induced by AMs.

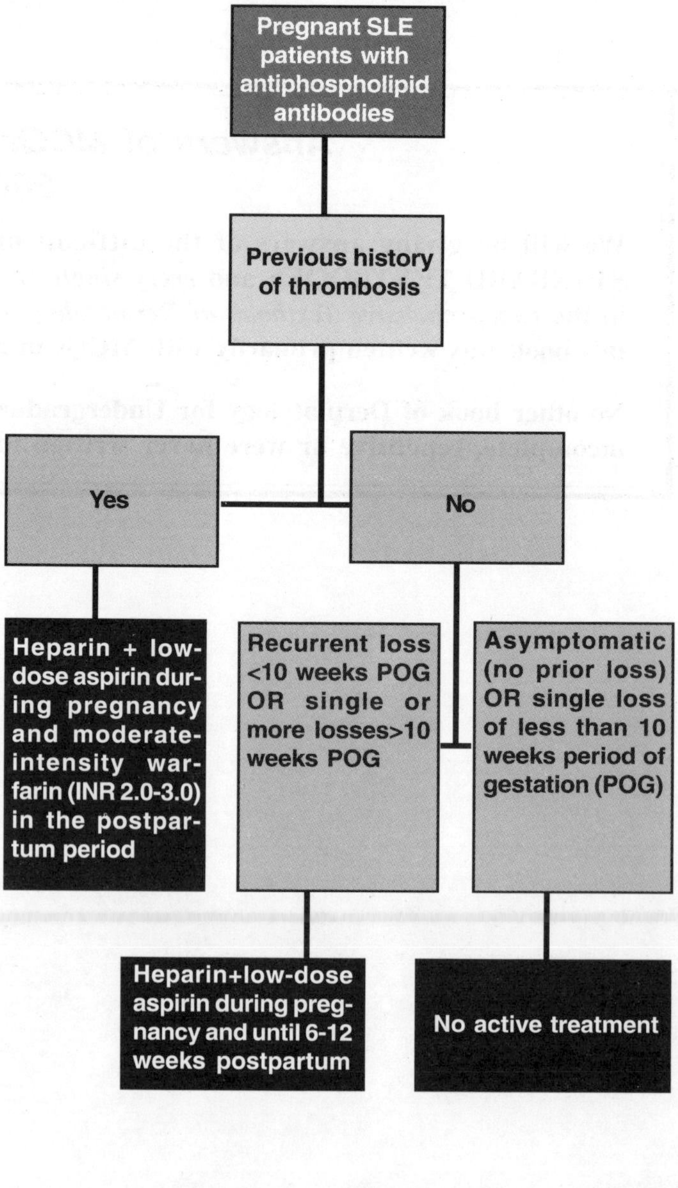

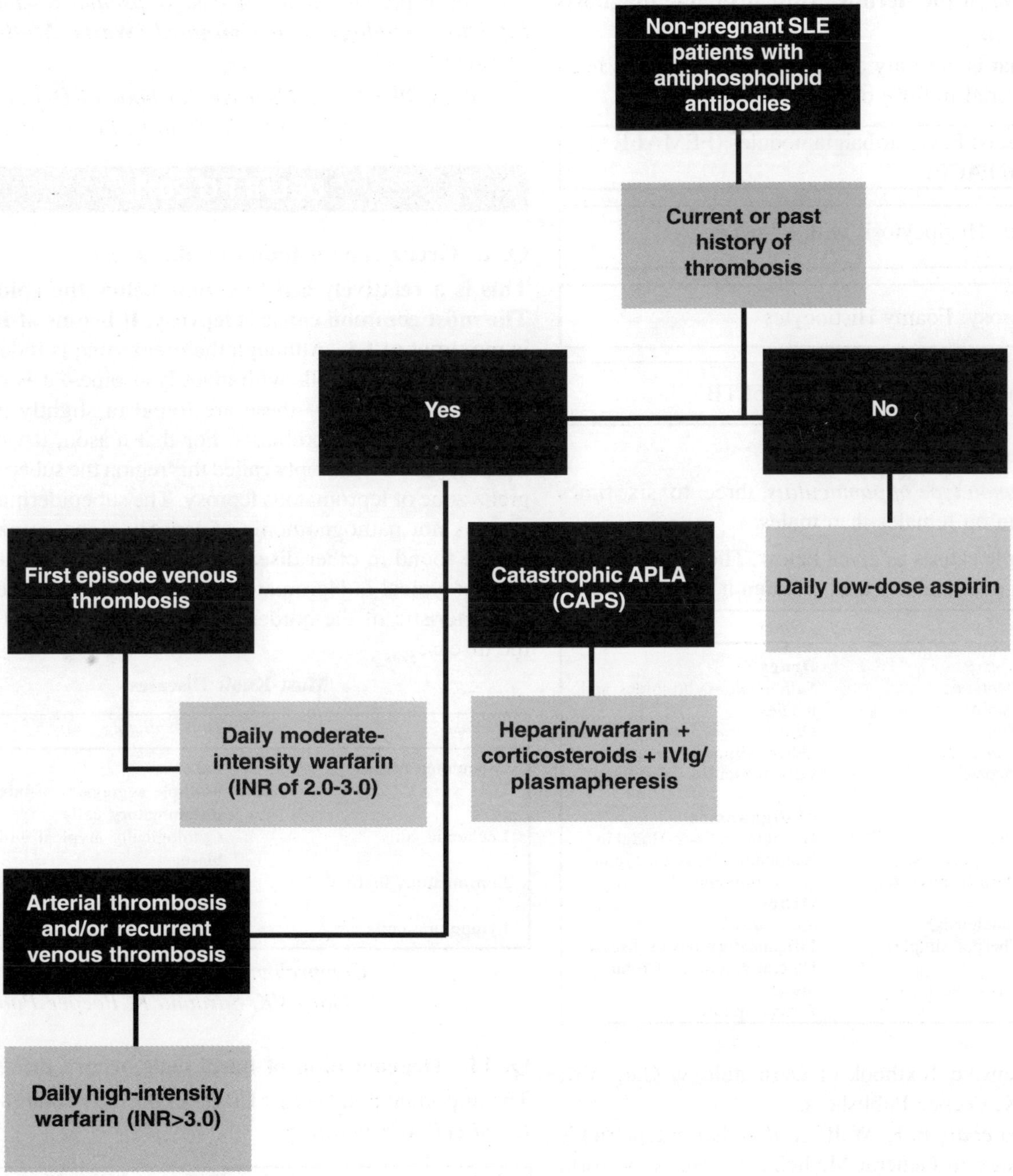

Reference: Harrison's Principles of Internal Medicine, Seventeenth Edition.

Q. 4. A young male presented with history of fever and a nodule in the leg. Histopathology of the nodule revealed foamy histiocytes and neutrophilic infiltrate in the dermis. Most probable diagnosis is?

This is a Q that is not only commonly asked but has been wrongly answered in 90% of guide books.

A.	• Sweets: Fever arthalgia nodules (FEMALE ON THE FACE)
B.	• Sinus Histiocytosis with LNpathy
C.	• Leprosy: Foamy Histiocytes
D.	• E indurativum: Tuberculide of TB

Erythema Nodosum

The most common type of panniculitis, three to six times more common on females than males.

It has multiple causes as given below. The most common cause in India in adults is TB in children it is Streptococci.

Infections	*Other*
Bacterial *Streptococcal infections*; *tuberculosis*, yersiniosis Other: *Salmonella, Campylobacter, Shigella,* brucellosis, psittacosis, *Mycoplasma*	**Drugs** *Sulfonamides;* bromides and iodides; *Oral contraceptives* Other: Minocycline, gold salts, penicillin, salicylates
Fungal Coccidioidomycosis, blastomycosis, histoplasmosis, sporotrichosis, dermatophytosis	**Malignancies** Hodgkin and non-Hodgkin lymphoma, leukemia, renal cell carcinoma
Viral Infectious mononucleosis, hepatitis B, orf, herpes simplex	**Other** *Sarcoidosis* Inflammatory bowel disease: Ulcerative colitis, Crohn disease Behcet disease
Other Amebiasis, giardiasis, ascariasis	

References:

1. Comprehensive Textbook of Dermatology: Garg VK, Sardana K, Peepee Publishers.
2. L Requena *et al.*, in K, Wolff *et al.* (eds.): Fitzpatrick's Dermatology in General Medicine,7th ed, New York, McGraw-Hill, 2008, 569–585.

Q. 5. This is seen in LP and of course arthiritis is not seen in LP.

Q. 6. Pseudoisomorphic phenomenon seen in:

The ***Koebner (isomorphic) phenomenon*** is defined as appearance of new lesions, identical to those in the diseased skin in the traumatized but otherwise normal skin. The Koebner reaction occurs in traumatized normal skin in ***vitiligo, psoriasis, and lichen planus (true)*** among other conditions. The Koebner phenomenon may occur in recent scars or at pressure point. In case of ***pseudo Koebners an infectious etiology is incriminated (Warts, Molluscum, Herpes).***

Page 29 : *Comprehensive Textbook of Dermatology: Garg VK, Sardana K, Peepee Publishers*

DELHI PG 2011

Q. 1. Grenz zone is found in all, *except:*

This is a relatively cell free zone below the epidermis. The most common cause is leprosy. It begins at BT and is maximal at LL. Although the grenz zone is indeed free of typical leprosy cells with giant lysosomes, it is not free from leprosy bacilli—these are found in slightly infested macrophages and fibroblasts. For that reason, it would be much clearer if we simply called this region the subepidermal grenz zone of lepromatous leprosy. The subepidermal grenz zone is not pathognomonic of leprosy since grenz zones can be found in other diseases as well. Whereas the grenz zone is typical in lepromatous leprosy, it is not necessarily characteristic of the borderline or the tuberculoid form of the disease.

Must Know Diseases

Disease	*Differentiating traits*
Granuloma faciale	Face Multiple aggregates of mixed inflammatory cells
Leukemia cutis	Cytologically atypical with blasts
Lepromatous leprosy	Numerous histiocytes with bubbly cytoplasm
Lymphoma cutis	Usually with B-cell lymphomas

Comprehensive Textbook of Dermatology: Garg VK, Sardana K, Peepee Publishers

Q. 14. Degeneration of basal cells occurs in:

The important point is that LP is *not the only condition with Basal cell degeneration.*

Disease	*Differentiating traits*
Fixed drug reaction	Lichenoid and deep perivascular mixed infiltrate with eosinophils, linear necrosis of basal cells
Graft-versus-host disease	Vacuolar change with scattered necrotic keratinocytes in epidermis and hair follicles-satellite cell necrosis

Contd.

Contd.

Lichen nitidus	Ball of lymphocytes and histiocytes in the dermis held by epidermal claw
Lichen planus	Lichenoid infiltrate, hyperkeratosis, hypergranulosis, saw-toothed base of acanthotic epidermis
Lichen striatus	Lichenoid and deep infiltrate that involves eccrine glands, scattered necrotic keratinocytes
Pityriasis lichenoides et varioliformis acuta	Parakeratosis, necrotic epidermis, extravasated RBCs, lichenoid and deep lymphocytic infiltrate

Comprehensive Textbook of Dermatology: Garg VK, Sardana K, Peepee Publishers

AIIMS MAY 2011

Ans. 1. (B)

There are two types of EB Acquired and Congenital.

The congenital has 3 types (Simplex, Junctional and Dystrophic)

A. Laminin 4 : Junctional

B. Collagen type 7: Dystrophic

C. Alpha 6 integrin: Junctional

D. Keratin 14: Simplex

Type gene	*Mutations*	*Locations*
Simplex		
Weber-Cockayne type	Keratins 5, 14	Hands, feet
Koebner type	Keratins 5, 14	Generalized
Dowling-Meara type	Keratins 5, 14	Generalized
Junctional		
Herlitz type	Laminin-5	Generalized, laryngeal
Generalized atrophic benign type	Type 17 collagen or Laminin A3, B3	Generalized
With pyloric atresia	$\alpha_6\beta_4$ integrin	Generalized, laryngeal, pylorus
Dystrophic		
Recessive type	Type 7 collagen	Generalized
Dominant types	Type 7 collagen	Generalized

Page 192/11 *Comprehensive Textbook of Dermatology: Garg VK, Sardana K, Peepee Publishers*

Ans. 2. (A) This is a Q of panniculitis

It is of two types: Septal and Lobular (see below). The most common is E Nodosum.

In this Q we have to basically differentiate between lobular and septal. Steroid induced panniculitis is a lobular panniculitis hence it is the answer.

For details please see below:

Classification of Panniculitis

Primary Panniculitis:

Septal	*Lobular*	*Combined Septal/ Lobular*
Erythema nodosum	Sclerema neonatorum	Nodular vasculitis/ erythema induratum
Erythema nodosum migrans/ subacute nodular migratory panniculitis	Subcutaneous fat necrosis of the newborn	Lupus erythematosus profundus/ connective tissue panniculitis
	Poststeroid panniculitis Cold panniculitis Foreign body/ factitial panniculitis Cytophagic histiocytic panniculitis (± septal) Pancreatic fat necrosis (± septal) Neutrophilic panniculitis/ subcutaneous Sweet's syndrome Weber-Christian disease	

SUBCUTANEOUS FAT NECROSIS OF THE NEWBORN

Clinical Presentation:

- Full-term infants upto six weeks of age.
- Asymptomatic, indurated, red to violaceous plaques and nodules.
- Predilection for buttocks, shoulders, cheeks and thighs.
- Resolves spontaneously in one to three months (usually without scarring).
- Rarely ulcerate and discharge milky material.
- Newborn has large body-surface-area-to-weight ratio.
- Greater saturated to unsaturated fatty acid ratio.
- Favors release of hydrolaces that induce breakdown of saturated fatty acids.
- Results in subcutaneous fat necrosis.

Clinicopathologic Correlation:

Clinical feature	*Pathologic feature*
Healthy infant with indurated plaque or nodule after birth trauma	Granulomatous lobular panniculitis with crystal formation in giant cells and lipocytes

SCLEREMA NEONATORUM

Clinopathologic Correlation:

Clinical feature	*Pathologic feature*
Premature neonate with waxy board-like induration	Septal thickening and fibrosis Expanded lobules and enlarged adipocytes

Differential Diagnosis:

Sclerema neonatorum	*Subcutaneous fat necrosis of the newborn*	*Poststeroid panniculitis*
Scant lobular inflammation	Mixed lobular inflammation	Presents in young children after discontinuing high-dose steroids without taper
Crystals seen only in lipocytes	Crystals seen in giant cells and lipocytes	Identical histologic features as subcutaneous fat necrosis

Page 20: *Comprehensive Textbook of Dermatology: Garg VK, Sardana K, Peepee Publishers*

Ans. 3. (D) This is a repeat Q and the answer is (D) as eye changes are seen in 30% of cases.

Page 261: *Comprehensive Textbook of Dermatology: Garg VK, Sardana K, Peepee Publishers*

Ans. 4. (A) The obvious answer is dementia which is classical of pellagra.

Acrodermatitis Enteropathica

Synonym: Zinc deficiency.

Major Points

- Classic presentation: Dermatitis, diarrhea, alopecia extreme irritability.
- Types:
  1. Genetic (autosomal recessive).
  2. Nutritional, found sporadically in premature and full-term infants.
  3. Endemically in the Middle East (growth failures and delayed pubertal maturation); caused by concurrent ingestion of high amounts of a zinc-binding ligand, phytate.
  4. Iatrogenic zinc deficiency associated with total parenteral nutrition.
- **Genetic form:** Usually occurs 1–2 weeks after weaning from breast feeding, and rarely during breast feeding; in bottle-fed infants it occurs 4–10 weeks of age.

Diagnosis

- Low plasma zinc levels are pathognomonic (blood must be collected in special acid-washed or plastic tubes).
- Low serum alkaline phosphatase (a zinc-dependent metalloenzyme).

Page 356: *Comprehensive Textbook of Dermatology: Garg VK, Sardana K, Peepee Publishers*

Ans. 5. (C)

Inflammatory Linear Verrucous Epidermal Nevus

Linear to curved, whorled (Blaschkoid) verrucous scaly plaques

Pruritic.

Lower extremity.

Occurs more frequently in children than in adults.

Can look identical to lichen striatus, but is persistent.

Ans. 6. (A)

The diagnosis is PWS and the answer is PDL (see below):

Lasers

Laser	*Wavelength (nm)*	*Type*	*Depth (μm)*	*Target*	*Usage*
CO_2	10,600	IR	20	Water	Resurface, destruction, coagulation cut
Erbium; YAG	2940	IR	1	Water	Superficial resurface, destruction
Holmium: YAG	2100	IR	200	Water	Superficial resurface, destruction
Nd: YAG	1064	IR	1600	Mel. Hb	Deep dermal pigment, black/blue tattoo, epilation non-ablative resurface, leg veins, telangiectasia
Diode	800,810,930	R	1400	Mel	Dermal pigment, epilation leg veins, vascular
Q-switched alexandrite	755	R	1300	Mel	Tattoo (black, blue, green) epilation pigmatation
Q-switched ruby	694	R	1200	Mel	Epidermal/Dermal pigment, tattoo (black, blue, green), epilation
Argon-pumped dye	630, 514, 488	O, G, B	600	Hb, mel	Vascular, epidermal pigment
PDL	585-595	Y	600	Hb, mel	Vascular, hypertrophic scar
Copper (bromide) vapor	578, 511	Y, G	400, 300	Hb, mel	Vascular, epidermal pigment
Krypton	568 531	Y G	400	Hb, mel	Vascular, epidermal pigment

Contd.

Contd.

Frequency doubled O-switched Nd: YAG/KTP	532	G	400	Mel, Hb	Vascular, epidermal pigment, red tattoo
Flash lamp pumped PDL	510	G	300	Mel, Hb	Vascular, hypertrophic scar
Argon	488, 514	B	200, 300	Mel, Hb	Vascular, epidermal pigment
Pulse excimer	351, 308, 193	UV	0.5	Protein	Psoriasis vitiligo, LASIK

IR: infrared; R: Red; O: Orange; Y: yellow; G: green; B: Blue; UV: Ultraviolet; Mel: Melanin; Hb: Hemoglobin

Page 435 : *Comprehensive Textbook of Dermatology: Garg VK, Sardana K, Peepee Publishers*

Ans. 7. (A)

This is a Q on Reticulate Pigmentary Disorders and the possible answer is A. All the other conditions have photosensitivity with immunodeficiency.

See the table below:

Dowling-Degos disease	Autosomal dominant, progressive symmetric bown macules, comedone-like follicular papules
Dohi	Acral location
Franceschetti–Jadassohn	Punctate pigment over waist, axilla, neck; hypohidrosis; palmoplantar keratosis; tooth, nail anomalies
Kitamura	Autosomal-dominant disorder; reticulated brown atrophic papules of distal extremities, palmar pits and breaks

Page 266: *Comprehensive Textbook of Dermatology: Garg VK, Sardana K, Peepee Publishers*

Ans. 8. (B)

Congenital varicella syndrome (fetal varicella syndrome or varicella embryopathy):

1. Fetal exposure ***before 20 weeks*** of gestation with greatest risk from 13 to 20 weeks.
2. 9% reported risk of developing disease with exposure.
3. Presents with dermatomal lesions: Denuded or scarred with associated underlying tissue hypoplasia.
4. Additional findings: Low birth weight, neurologic (e.g. hydrocephalus, retardation, seizures), ophthalmologic (e.g., chorioretinitis, cataracts, nystagmus), musculoskeletal (e.g., extremity hypoplasia and paresis), gastrointestinal and genitourinary anomalies.

Intrauterine Exposure

1. Varicella zoster immunoglobulin (VZIG) given within 5 days to non-immune mothers with recent VZV exposure.
2. Acyclovir is considered safe for pregnant women who are infected and may minimize the risk of disease in the newborn.

Neonatal Varicella

1. Due to *fetal exposure near the time of delivery* with maternal infection between 5 days prior to and 2 days following delivery.
2. 23-62% risk of developing disease with exposure.
3. Cutaneous findings from 1 to 16 days postpartum: papulovesicular lesions which can become hemorrhagic or necrotic.

   High risk for disseminated disease pneumonitis, hepatitis, encephalitis.

Neonatal Varicella

1. VZIG.
2. Acyclovir.
3. Isolation.

Infantile Herpes Zoster

1. Develops during first year of life after in utero varicella exposure.
2. 2% of infants exposed to intrauterine varicella will develop infantile herpes zoster.
3. Clinical findings: Papulovesicles in dermatomal pattern, typically thoracic area.

Infantile Herpes Zoster

1. No specific therapy needed if immunocompetent.
2. Consider systemic acyclovir, especially if there are hemorrhagic or disseminated lesions.

AIIMS NOVEMBER–DECEMBER 2010

Q. 1. A teen age girl with moderate acne also complaining of irregular menses. Drug of choice will be:

The most important point is that with this history there is *no proof of a hyperandrogenic defect*. Merely having an irregular menses does not prove a androgenic defect. Secondly **CPA IS NEVER GIVEN ALONE IN ACNE. It is always given as an OCP.**

Hormonal Treatments

This form of therapy is recommended for cases where the standard antibiotic regimens fails, menstrual control and/ or contraception is required with acne therapy (isotretinoin use) and where oral isotretinoin is inappropriate or not available.

Antiandrogens Vs Isotretinoin

It has been our experience as of other authors (Larsen TH *et al.*) that the best drug remains isotretinoin (85 ± 10% improvement), followed by tetracycline (54 ± 3%) and the OCP of CPA plus ethinyl oestradiol (65 ± 4% improvement). Hormonal therapy is an option only in case where acne is not responding to conventional therapy. In all other case isotretinoin is a preferred drug. Even case with normal serum androgen respond well to hormonal therapy.

Reference:

- 42.50 Chapter 42: Disorders of the Sebaceous Glands: Rooks Textbook of Dermatology, 8th edition.

Q. 2. Malignant pustule is seen in:

Cutaneous Anthrax

It is caused by Bacillus anthracis a gram-positive, spore-forming bacillus that derives its name from the Greek word for coal or charcoal, anthrakos.

Clinical features:In more than 95% of cases of endemic disease, spores are transmitted from infected animals or their products by means of skin abrasions. A pruritic macule or papule appears at the site of inoculation. The primary lesion progresses to a vesicle or a bulla after 24-48 hours. The bulla enlarges to 1-2 cm, spontaneously ruptures, and forms an ulcer. A hemorrhagic crust develops and is often accompanied by striking edema. *The edema is also referred to a "malignant pustule" which is a misnomer.*

Reference:

- **Page No. 48**: Anthrax : Comprehensive Textbook of Dermatology : Garg VK, Sardana K, Peepee Publishers.

Q. 3. Chemical peeling is done by *all except*:

A. Trichloroacetic acid
B. Phosphoric acid
C. Carboxylic acid
D. Kojic acid

This Q is most likely wrongly framed wrong or the reverse as chemical peeling is done by *only TCA in the Q.*

Chemical Peel

Chemical peel produces a controlled partial thickness injury to the skin. Following the insult to the skin, a wound healing process ensues that can regenerate epidermis from surrounding epithelium and adnexal structures, decrease solar elastosis, and replace and reorient the new dermal connective tissue. The result is an improved clinical appearance of the skin, with fewer rhytides and decreased pigmentary dyschromia.

Peeling Agents

1. Glycolic acid.
2. Jessner's solution.
3. Pyruvic acid.
4. Resorcinol.
5. Salicylic acid.
6. Trichloracetic acid.

Reference:

- **Page No. 481:** TB: Comprehensive Textbook of Dermatology : Garg VK, Sardana K, Peepee Publishers.

Q. 4. Farmer with single verrucous plaque on leg. Which of the following could be the lesion?

A.	• Verruca vulgaris: Viral wart is small and is not only seen in farmers
B.	• TBVC
C.	• Mycetom: Can be seen in farmers but it is not verrucous, it has nodules and sinuses
D.	• LPH: Itchy, violaceous

Definition: It's a verrucous (wart like) form of reinfection tuberculosis.

Syn warty tuberculosis, prosectors wart, verruca-necrogenica, tuberculosis cutis verruca, postprimary inoculation tuberculosis and verrucous tuberculosis.

It occurs when the skin of a previously infected or BCG-immunized host, possessing a ***moderate or high degree of immunity***, is subjected to exogenous reinfection. Reinoculation occurs at sites of minor abrasions or wounds. It commonly occurs in physicians, pathologists, medical students, laboratory attendants, veterinarians, ***farmers,*** and butchers (tuberculous cattle). Autoinoculation from tuberculous sputum (rare).

Reference:

- **Page No. 66:** TB: Comprehensive Textbook of Dermatology: Garg VK, Sardana K, Peepee Publishers.

Q. 5. 25 years old labourer 3 years back presented with penile ulcer not treated. Later he presented with neurological symptoms for which he got treated. Test to monitor response to treatment is:

VDRL

Cardiolipin (Non-treponemal) Tests:Venereal Diseases Research Laboratory (VDRL) is the best test for *monitoring therapy in India*. A titer of > 1:8 is positive and a titre <1:8 is a False Positive VDRL. The other tests for follow up of therapy include VDRL, IgM-FTA-ABS, IgM-ELISA.

Reference:

- **Page No. 106:** Syphilis : Comprehensive Textbook of Dermatology : Garg VK, Sardana K, Peepee Publishers.

AIIMS MAY 2010

Q. 1. Which of the following is not true about lepromin test?

A.	• It is used to diagnose cases but is not a specific test as it indicates only exposure to the disease
B.	• Yes because the immune response takes time to develop
C.	• It is used only for Ridley Jopling classification
D.	• The last statement is not untrue but this does not always happen

References:

- Comprehensive Textbook of Dermatology: Garg VK, Sardana K, Peepee Publishers.
- **Hastings:** Textbook of Leprosy, 1998.

  How to Diagnose and Treat Leprosy ILEP.

  How to Recognize and Manage Leprosy Reactions ILEP.

  Report of the Eighth Meeting of the WHO Technical Advisory Group on Leprosy Control Aberdeen, Scotland 21st April, 2006,WHO.

Q. 2. Leprosy affects all of the following *except*:

The answer of this question depends on the options.The organs that are *rarely* involved include the following:

Organs with none or minimal degree of infiltration or dysfunction	
Brain	Striated muscle
Cerebellum	Ureter
Leptomeninges	Bladder
Spinal cord	Urethra
Pancreas	Prostate
Lungs	Seminal vesicles
Heart	External genitalia
Great vessels	Breasts
Gallbladder	Vagina
Pancreas	Uterus
Esophagus	Ovaries
Stomach	Thyroid gland
Small intestine	Parathyroid gland
Large intestine	Pituitary gland
Striated muscle	Pineal gland

Of these ***CNS is never involved*** of the rest the CVS and ovary are less commonly involved. The issue is of Lung Vs Ovary/Endometrium. Lung is usually more involved than the ovary and endometrium is more involved than the ovary. This is because the spread of leprosy inside the body is primarily by vascular spread and the vascular supply of the lung and enometrium is more than the ovary. Moreover if ovary involvement is more than that of endometrium leprosy being common in India would be a leading cause of infertility which it is not table is given below which details the lung involvement.

Table: Lung involvement
Lower respiratory tract
Larger bronchial infiltration (uncommon)[2,20]
Lung parenchyma sparing [2,8,10,20]
Minimal cellular infiltration of lungs[75,209]
AFB in alveolar walls[1]
Pulmonary tuberculosis[1, 4, 21-24]
Bronchopneumonia[1, 3, 5]
Corpulmonale (rare) (due to pulmonary embolism in erythema nodosum leprosum)[210]
Amyloid deposition in the lung (rare)[3, 5]
Female reproductive system
Female genital tract spared[3]
Mild infiltrates in vaginal membranes, endometrial walls, uterine walls and fallopian tubes[75]
Ovaries spared[63, 75, 141]
Ovaries involved[118]
Uterine and ovarian atrophy[6]
Normal menarche, menstruation, fertility and menopause[144]

References:

- Visceral Leprosy. Int J of Dermatology 2000, 39, 641-48.

- Comprehensive Textbook of Dermatology. Garg Sardana Peepee Publishers.
- **Hastings:** Textbook of Leprosy, 1998.

Q. 6. This is a Q that has been asked previously and focuses on Neutrophilic Dermatoses.

Fever, Arthralgia

Male/Female		Female face
Shins **E Nodosum**	**Leprosy** **ENT**	**Sweet's syndrome**

Weber-Christian disease: *Uncommon* idiopathic lobular panniculitis (ILP). It is seen in *females* 30-60 years of age. Involves the the thighs and lower legs.

Causes of panniculitis

a. ***Panniculitis (with vasculitis)***
   - PAN, nodular **Vasculitis,** Churg-Strauss syndrome.
   - Mixed.
     Traumatic, histiocytic cytophagic type.

b. ***Panniculitis (without vasculitis)***
   i. *Septal*
      - Erythema Nodosum.
      - S/C Gr Annulare, scleroderma.

   ii. *Lobular*
      - Lymphocyte=Lupus
      - Eosinophil=Eosinophilic fascitis
      - Histiocyte=Cytophagic histiocytic panniculitis
      - Foam cells=Weber Christian disease.

Reference:

- **Page 23:** Comprehensive Textbook of Dermatology: Garg VK, Sardana K, Peepee Publishers.

Q. 9. Angioedema is merely swelling of the mucosa which could be either acquired and associated with urticaria or without urticaria. Hereditary angioedema is associated with lesions without wheals.

It is important to know the investigations required for diagnosis of angioedema.

Angioedema without wheals

Basic tests	*Advanced tests*	*Diagnosis*
Low C4 Levels	C1 inh levels (Reduced by 30%-50%) C1 inh function (N)	Type I HAE
	Normal C1 inh levels C1 inh function (decreased)	Type II HAE
	C1 inh levels (low) C1 inh function(decreased) C1q (low)	Acquired AE Type 1: Underlying malignancy Type 2:Antibody to C1 inh
NormalC4 levels	Drug history	Drug induced, e.g. ACEI
	Genetic testing	Oestrogen dependent angioedema (Type III HAE)
	Peripheral blood count: eosinophilia	Gleich syndrome
	NAD	Idiopathic

References:

- **Rook's Textbook of Dermatology**, 8th ed./edited by Tony Burns, Stephen Breathnach, Neil Cox Christopher Griffiths.
- **Fitzpatrick's Dermatology in General Medicine,** Seventh edition, Klaus Wolff, Lowell A. Goldsmith, Stephen I. Katz, MD, Barbara A. Gilchrest, Amys. Paller, David I. Leffell, Tata McGraw Hill, 2008.

AIIMS NOVEMBER 2009

Q. 2. Treatment of choice in genital wart in pregnancy:

A.	• Salicyclic/Lactic acid is probably the best option for non genital warts
B.	• This is not available in India and is an extract of podophyllin which is a DOC for vulval warts but is an abortifacient
C.	• Imiquimod IS NOT SAFE IN PREGNANCY*
D.	• Safest therapy is TCA 90%, Cryotherapy and Surgery

* This is a mistake perpetuated by guide books and certain books in the Indian market. (CDC Guidelines for STD "The safety of imiquimod during pregnancy has not been established.")

Imiquimod, sinecatechins, podophyllin and podofilox should ***not be used during pregnancy***. Genital warts can proliferate and become friable during pregnancy. Although removal of warts during pregnancy can be considered, resolution might be incomplete or poor until pregnancy is complete. Rarely, HPV types 6 and 11 can cause respiratory papillomatosis in infants and children, although the route of transmission (i.e., transplacental, perinatal, or postnatal) is not completely understood. Whether cesarean section prevents respiratory papillomatosis in infants and children also is unclear. *Cesarean delivery* is indicated for women with genital warts if the pelvic outlet is obstructed or if vaginal delivery would result in excessive bleeding. Pregnant women with genital warts should be counselled concerning the low risk for warts on the larynx (recurrent respiratory papillomatosis) in their infants or children.

References:

- Sexually Transmitted Diseases Treatment Guidelines, 2010 CDC USA.
- Comprehensive Textbook of Dermatology: Garg VK, Sardana K, Peepee Publishers.

Q. 8. As vasculitis is a common Q asked a simple table to enable diagnosis is given below:

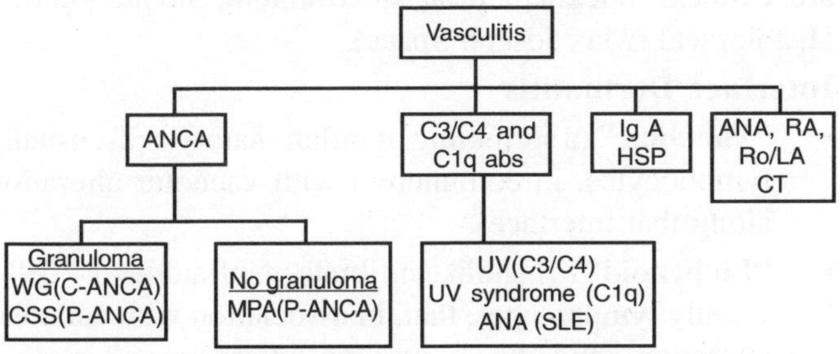

Table: Basic diagnostic protocol based on clinical findings and relevant investigations

Clinical findings	*Tests*	*Diagnosis*
Drugs, URTI	Not needed	**Cutaneous**
Environmental agents		**Leukocytoclastic**
(No Visceral Disease)		**Vasculitis**
Child with purpura	Vascular deposit of IgA	**Henoch-Schönlein Purpura**
Urticaria	Assess	
	C3/C4 and C1q abs	**Urticarial Vasculitis (UV)**
		SLE
	1. C3/C4: Normal	1. Normo-complementemic UV2
	2. C3/C4: Low	2. Hypo-complementemic UV3
	3. Anti C1q abs	3. UV syndrome 4
	4. SLE	4. Lupus vasculitis
Visceral disease, Renal	**ANCA (+)**	
Pulmonary, GIT involvement and nephropathy	1. Granulomatous inflammation	**Wegener's granulomatosis**
	2. Asthma, eosinophilia granulomatous inflammation	**Churg-Strauss syndrome**
	3. No granuloma	**Microscopic polyangitis**
Visceral disease, renal	**(+) ANA, RF, Anti DNA**	**CT vasculitis**
Pulmonary, GIT involvement and nephropathy	**RoLA, ACA, RF**	
Sclerosis, dry eye, arthritis or cutaneous lupus		
Nodules, livedo acral gangrene and/or neuropathy	NA	**PAN**
High grade fever	Blood culture and murmur	**Septic vasculitis**
Recurrent purpura, hematuria	Hematological abnormality	**Paraneoplastic vasculitis**
Recalcitrant to therapy	Mass on imaging	

References:

- **Rook's Textbook of Dermatology**, 8th ed., edited by Tony Burns, Stephen Breathnach, Neil Cox Christopher Griffiths.
- **Fitzpatrick's Dermatology in General Medicine,** 7th ed., Klaus Wolff, Lowell A. Goldsmith, Stephen I. Katz, MD, Barbara A. Gilchrest, Amys. Paller, David I. Leffell, Tata McGraw Hill 2008.
- Comprehensive Textbook of Dermatology: Garg VK, Sardana K, Peepee Publishers.

UPSC 2010

Q. 3. As this is a very commonly asked Q. The Features are given below. The features in Bold have been asked as MCQ in various exams.

Congenital Syphilis

Early congenital syphilis (within first 2 years of life)

- Failure to thrive.

- Mucosal lesions: ***Snuffles.***
- Skin lesions:
  - They mimic ***secondary syphilis*** and heal with rhagades.
  - Bullous eruption of palms and soles can be seen (***syphilitic pemphigus***).
  - Condylomata lata can be seen around the anus and genitalia.
  - There is sparse hair and brittle, atrophic nails.
- Hepatosplenomegaly and moderate generalized lymphadenopathy may occur.
- Osteochondritis and later periostitis especially of the long bones (may present as ***pseudoparalysis***).
- Others: These include *meningitis*, nephrotic syndrome, *choroidoretinitis*, anaemia and thrombocytopenia.

Late congenital syphilis (after 2 years of age)

Mimic accelerated late stage acquired syphilis (though the cardiovascular system is usually spared). The various features can be classified under two heads:

1. **Inflammatory:**
   - ***Interstitial keratitis (most common late feature 20-50%).***
   - Deafness (otolabyrinthitis).
   - ***Clutton's joints*** (bilateral painless effusion of the knee joints).
   - Gummata of nasal septum, palate and throat; skin and bone (as in acquired syphilis).
   - Neurosyphilis (seizures, mental deficiency, juvenile tabes dorsalis and general paralysis).
   - Paroxysmal cold haemoglobinuria.
2. **Malformations:**
   - **Facies:** There is ***frontal bossing, bulldog appearance*** (hypoplastic maxilla, high arched palate and prominent mandible); ***saddle-nose and circumoral rhagades.***
   - **Dental anomalies:** These include:
     - ***Hutchinson's incisors***: The ***upper central incisors*** are conical, tapered towards the apex and notched. This can be associated with the Hutchinson's triad (Hutchinson's incisors, interstitial keratitis and nerve deafness.)
     - Moon's (Mulberry) molars (1st lower molars are dome shaped with hypoplastic cusps.)
   - **Skeletal signs:** These include bony sclerosis (generalized) or nodules (localized). Long bones are primarily affected especially the tibia with anterior bowing (***sabre tibia).***

References:

- Comprehensive Textbook of Dermatology: Garg VK, Sardana K, Peepee Publishers.
- Sexually Transmitted Diseases, King Holmes, P. Sparling, Walter Stamm, Peter Piot, Judith Wasserheit, Lawrence Corey, Myron Cohen 4 2007, **McGraw-Hill Companies.**

Q. 6. The earliest sensation to be lost in leprosy is:

"The type C fibers which mediate sensations towards heat and cold or different temperatures are lost first before loss of pain or light touch fibres. This is preceded by decreased sweating and in some cases, eventuates into anhidrosis on the palms or soles, suggesting involvement of the sympathetic nerves."

DELHI PG FEBRUARY 2010

Q. 4. The most characteristic finding in lichen planus is:

This is a commonly wrongly answered Q. It must be emphasized that BCD is not diagnostic of LP. It can be seen in various conditions.The pathognomic findings of LP are: Clinical: Wickham Stria, Nail (thinning and pterygium), Histological (Max Joseph Space).

Interface Dermatitis

- **"Vacuolar"** (a sprinkling of inflammatory cells, usually lymphocytes, in conjunction with vacuolar alteration along that interface).
- **"Lichenoid"** (a bandlike infiltrate of inflammatory cells, usually lymphocytes, that, in association with vacuolar alteration, tends to obscure the interface).

  Examples:
  - Apoptic cells–Erythema multiforme.
  - Minimal apotopsis–Dermatomyositis.
  - Variable–Drug eruption.
  - BMZ thickening–LE.

Reference:

- **Page 22:** Comprehensive Textbook of Dermatology: Garg VK, Sardana K, Peepee Publishers.

Q. 6. Erythema multiforme is associated with:

Etiology

A cutaneous reaction to a variety of antigenic stimuli, most commonly to herpes simplex.

Infection: Especially following herpes simplex, *Mycoplasma.*

Drugs: Sulfonamides, phenytoin, barbiturates, phenylbutazone, penicillin, allopurinol.

Idiopathic: Probably also due to undetected herpes simplex or *Mycoplasma.*

Skin Lesions: Dull red. Iris or targetlike lesions. Localized to hands and face or generalized

Sites of Predilection: Dorsa of hands, palms and soles; forearms; feet; face; elbows and knees; penis (50%) and vulva.

Mucous Membranes: Erosions with fibrin membranes; occasionally ulcerations: lips, oropharynx, nasal, conjunctival, vulvar, anal.

Other Organs: Eyes, with corneal ulcers, anterior uveitis.

References:

- **Fitzpatrick's Dermatology in General Medicine,** Seventh Edition, Klaus Wolff, Lowell A. Goldsmith, Stephen I. Katz, MD, Barbara A. Gilchrest, Amys. Paller, David I. Leffell, Tata McGraw Hill 2008.
- Comprehensive Textbook of Dermatology: Garg VK, Sardana K, Peepee Publishers.

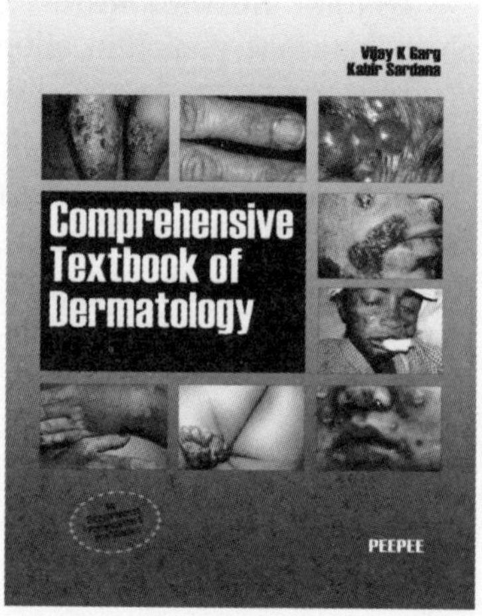

Part II

Chapter-wise MCQs
(Based on Comprehensive Textbook of Dermatology)
It is to be noted that all the MCQs asked in the last 2 years after the launch of the book have come from the Comprehensive Textbook of Dermatology

How to use	*Chapters that are important*	*Exams relevant*
The page numbers correspond to the textbook. Those students who have the book can cross-verify. † *Important MCQs* †† *Most Important MCQs* ††† *Extremely Important MCQs*	Introduction Infections Infestations STD HIV Allergic diseases Bullous disorders Papulosquamous Pigmented disorders Therapy	AIIMS PGI UPSC USMLE

Section 1

INTRODUCTION OF SKIN DISEASES*

1. The distribution of keratins (K) in the basal layers is: †

A. K5/K14 B. K1/K10
C. K2/K11 D. K6/K16

2. Cholesterol sulfate is found in which layer of the skin?

A. S corneum B. S lucidum
C. S basale D. None of the above

3. Total cell turnover time is: †

A. 28 days B. 40 days
C. 52 days D. 14 days

4. Which part of the hair is functionally fixed?

A. Isthmus B. Stem
C. Bulb D. Adamson fringe

5. Apocrine miliaria is a name given to which of the following conditions? †

A. Fox-Fordyce disease
B. Hidradenitis suppurativa
C. Fordyce's spots
D. Tyson's glands

6. Epidermal melanin unit has a ratio of: †

A. 10:1 B. 32:1
C. 1:10 D. 36:1

7. Tennis racquet shaped granules are seen in which cell? †

A. Melanocyte B. Langerhans cell
C. Macrophage D. Lymphocyte

8. Match the following antigens with the diseases:

A. Keratins 5 and 14 a. DH
B. Laminin 5 b. P. vulgaris
C. Desmoglein 3 c. Junctional EB
D. Transglutaminase 2 d. EB simplex

9. Acantholysis is seen in all *except:* †

A. Dermatitis herpetiformis
B. Pemphigus
C. Leprosy
D. Impetigo

10. Match the following:

A. Naked tubercle a. Leprosy
B. Tuberculoid granulomas b. Sarcoidosis
C. Palisaded c. Granuloma annulare
D. Suppurative d. Hidradenitis suppurativa

11. Ballooning degeneration is classic of: †

A. Herpes B. Acid burn
C. Thermal burn D. Leprosy

12. Match the split in the following:

A. Suprabasal a. Pemphigus
B. Intraspinous b. Impetigo
C. Subcorneal c. PCT
D. Subepidermal d. Herpes

13. Match the stains with the tissue/organism:

A. Fontana-Masson a. Elastic fibers
B. Periodic Acid-Schiff (PAS) b. Collagen
C. Verhoeff-van Gieson c. Melanocyte
D. Masson trichrome d. Fungi

14. Match the following:

A. S-100 a. Follicular B-cell lymphoma
B. HMB-45 b. Nerve
C. Bcl6 c. Melanocyte
D. CEA d. Paget's

15. Which is the classic lesion of urticaria?

A. Macule B. Papule
C. Nodule D. Wheal

16. What is the level of the burrow in scabies? †

A. Epidermis B. Dermis
C. S corneum D. S spinosum

17. Match the following:

A. Dimple sign a. Sarcoidosis
B. Darier's sign b. Mastocytosis
C. Auspitz's sign c. Psoriasis
D. Diascopy d. Dermatofibroma

18. All of the following fluoresce green *except*:

A. Tinea capitis
B. Kerion
C. Erythrasma
D. Pseudomonas

* **Pages 1-29:** Comprehensive Textbook of Dermatology, Garg VK, Sardana K.

19. Patch test is best read at: †

A. 1 day
B. 2 days
C. 3 days
D. 4 days

20. Acet whitening test is done for:

A. Molluscum
B. Acne
C. Tinea capitis
D. Genital warts

Answers :

1. A	2. A	3. C	4. A
5. A	6. D	7. B	8. Ad,Bc,Cb,Da
9. C,A	10. Ab,Ba,Cc,Dd	11. A	12. Aa,Bd,Cb,Dc
13. Ac,Bd,Ca,Db	14. Ab,Bc,Ca,Dd	15. D	16. C
17. Ad,Bb,Cc,Da	18. C	19. D	20. D

Section 2

INFECTIONS*

1. Dose of acyclovir for herpes genitalis is: †

A. 200 mg 5 times a day
B. 400 mg 5 times a day
C. 800 mg 5 times a day
D. Topical acyclovir

2. Best treatment for H zoster is: †

A. Oral acyclovir 800 mg 5 times/day
B. Valaciclovir 1 gm TDS
C. Famciclovir 250 mg TDS × 7 to 10 days
D. Topical acyclovir

3. Match the following:

A. Nasal vestibule — a. Coryneforms
B. Toe clefts — b. S. aureus
C. External ear — c. Aspergillus
D. Axilla — d. Brevibacterium

4. Stuck on crust, appearance is classical of: †

A. Impetigo
B. Folliculitis
C. Furuncle
D. Carbuncle

5. Which of the following correlates with cutaneous streptococcal infection? †

A. ASLO
B. NADase
C. DNAase B
D. Grams stain

6. Ofuji disease is also known as:

A. Pseudofolliculitis barbae
B. Bockharts impetigo
C. Sycosis barbae
D. Eosinophilic folliculitis

7. Pastia lines are seen in: †

A. Scarlet fever
B. Leprosy
C. Impetigo
D. Pseudomonas

8. Corynebacterium causes all of the following *except:*†

A. Erythrasma
B. Malakoplakia
C. Pitted keratolysis
D. Trichomycosis axillaris

9. Match the following:

A. Tinea nigra — a. Malassezia furfur
B. White piedra — b. Piedra hortae
C. Tinea versicolor — c. Trichosporum ovoides
D. Black piedra — d. Phaeoannellomyces werneckii

10. A child came with a boggy swelling on the scalp with loss of hair. This is caused by zoophilic species. Name it. †

A. T mentagrophytes
B. M canis
C. T verrucosum
D. T rubrum

11. A child came with alopecia with scutulae, what is the possible diagnosis? †

A. Grey patch
B. Kerion
C. Favus
D. Black dot

12. T tonsurans causes which type of tinea capitis? †

A. Grey patch
B. Kerion
C. Favus
D. Black dot

13. Which of the following is the drug of choice for tinea capitis?

A. Griseofulvin
B. Terbinafine
C. Itraconazole
D. Fluconazole

14. Linear eruption of nodules along the lymphatics following trauma on the distal extremity in a gardener is treated by: †

* **Pages 30-69:** MUST READ Comprehenive Textbook of Dermatology, Garg VK, Sardana K (most important is Fungal Infections).

A. Terbinafine	B. Itraconazole
C. Fluconazole	D. KI

15. Match the following:

A. Sporotrichosis	a. South America
B. Chromoblastomycosis	b. Asteroid bodies
C. Lobomycosis	c. Medlar bodies
D. Cryptococcosis	d. India ink

Answers :

1. A	**2. B**	**3. Ab,Bd,Cc,Da**	**4. A**
5. C	**6. D**	**7. A**	**8. B**
9. Ad,Bc,Ca,Db	**10. B**	**11. C**	**12. D**
13. A	**14. D**	**15. Ab,Ba,Cc,Dd**	

INSECT BITES AND INFESTATIONS*

1. A child comes in summer with papules, with a central haemorrhagic punctum on exposed parts of the body. What is the likely diagnosis? †

A. Insect bite RTN	B. PMLE
C. Solar urticaria	D. PCT

2. Kissing lesions are characteristic of all *except:*

A. Beetle dermatitis	B. Primary chancre
C. Chancroid	D. PMLE

3. A child has scalp pruritus with enlarged cervical lymph nodes, what is the diagnosis? †

A. Tinea capitis	B. Pediculosis
C. Lichen planus	D. Psoriasis

4. Plica polonica is a complication seen in: †

A. Tinea capitis	B. Pediculosis
C. Lichen planus	D. Psoriasis

5. Match the following: †

A. Vagabond disease	a. Pediculosis capitis
B. Maculae cerulae	b. Altered blood
C. STD	c. Pediculosis pubis
D. Cotrimoxazole	d. Pediculosis corporos

6. Match the following:

A. Nodular scabies	a. Crusted scabies
B. Highly infectious	b. Steroid
C. Palm and sole	c. Childhood scabies
D. Scabies incognito	d. Steroid

7. Match the following: †

A. Gamma benzene hexachloride	a. Contraindicated in pregnancy
B. Permethrin cream 5%	b. Pediculosis
C. Permethrin cream 1%	c. Scabies
D. Sulfur ointment	d. Infant

8. Match the following:

A. Larva currens	a. Ancylostoma-braziliensis
B. Diethyl (Diethyl) carbamazine	b. Filariasis
C. Albendazole 400 mg	c. Pinworm
D. Cutaneous larva migrans	d. Strongyloides

Answers :

1. A	**2. D**	**3. B**	**4. B**
5. Ad,Bb, Cc,Da	**6. Ad,Ba, Cc,Db**	**7. Aa,Bc, Cb,Dd**	**8. Ad,Bb, Cc,Da**

SEXUALLY TRANSMITTED DISEASES**

1. A male comes with multiple painful ulcers, what is the most likley diagnosis? †

A. Chancre	B. Chancroid
C. Herpes	D. Aphthosis

2. The bubo in chancroid is: †

A. Painful	B. Unilateral
C. Multilocular	D. Painless

3. Culture medium used for chancroid is all *except:*†

A. Blood agar
B. Enriched blood agar
C. Chocolate agar
D. Mc Coy cell line

4. Most sensitive test to diagnose chancroid is: †

A. Culture	B. Biopsy
C. Smear	D. PCR

5. The therapy of chancroid is all *except:* †

A. Azithromycin 1 g orally in a single dose
B. Ceftriaxone 250 mg intramuscularly (IM) in a single dose
C. Ciprofloxacin 500 mg orally twice a day for 3 days
D. Penicillin injection

* **Pages 81-86:** MUST READ Comprehensive Textbook of Dermatology: Garg VK, Sardana K, Peepee Publishers.
** **Extremely important** MUST READ **Pages 88-106** Comprehensive Textbook of Dermatology, Garg VK, Sardana K, Peepee Publishers. Also see Guidelines of STD by NACO and CDC.†

6. The therapy of chancroid in pregnancy is: †

A. Azithromycin 1 g orally in a single dose
B. Ciprofloxacin 500 mg orally twice a day for 3 days
C. Doxycycline
D. Septran

7. The most common form of herpes genitalis is:

A. Asymptomatic
B. Initial episode
C. Primary infection
D. Recurrent episode

8. The viral shedding in primary stage of herpes is for:

A. 1 week B. 2 weeks
C. 3 weeks D. 4 weeks

9. A patient of herpes has 7 episodes in a year which of the following will be the drug of choice? †

A. Acyclovir 400 mg orally three times a day for 7-10 days
B. Famciclovir 250 mg orally three times a day for 7-10 days
C. Acyclovir 400 mg orally twice a day
D. Famciclovir 250 mg orally twice a day

10. Which of the following are given in a thymidine kinase resistant mutant? †

A. Foscarnet, 40 mg/kg
B. Cidofovir gel 1%
C. Famciclovir
D. Valaciclovir

11. Friable, bleeding ulcers are seen in:

A. Syphilis
B. Chancroid
C. Granuloma inguinale
D. Herpes

12. In a patient of donovaniosis with HIV + which of the following drugs are to be added? †

A. Azithromycin B. Ceftriaxone
C. Gentamicin D. Penicillin

13. All are seen in LGV *except:*

A. Sign of groove
B. Vesicle
C. Esthimene
D. Pseudobubo

14. A male comes with a single painless ulcer in how many weeks will it heal spontaneously?

A. 1 week B. 2 weeks
C. 3 weeks D. 6 weeks

15. Which is the most sensitive test to diagnose primary chancre? †††

A. VDRL B. DG
C. TPHA D. FTAbs

16. Which is the most specific test to diagnose primary chancre? †††

A. VDRL B. DG
C. TPHA D. FTAbs

17. The most infectious lesion of syphilis is:

A. Primary chancre B. C lata
C. Mucus patch D. Rash

18. A man who is VDRL + has dementia with delusion of grandeur, what is the diagnosis?

A. Neurosyphilis
B. Gumma
C. General paralysis of insane (GPI)
D. Tabes dorsalis (TD)

19. Match the following:

A. Snuffles	a. Tabes dorsalis
B. Clutton joint	b. Skin
C. Gumma	c. Child
D. Charcot's joints	d. Nose

20. Match the following:

A. Higoumenaki sign	a. Osteochondritis
B. Pemphigus syphilitica	b. Late stage
C. Paroxysmal cold	c. Bulla on palm and sole haemoglobinuria
D. Parrot's pseudoparalysis	d. Clavicle

21. All of the following are used to monitor therapy *except:* †

A. DG B. IgM-FTA-ABS
C. IgM-ELISA D. VDRL

22. Which of the following is used for diagnosis of syphilis? ††

A. VDRL > 1:4 B. VDRL > 1:6
C. VDRL > 1:8 D. VDRL > 1:2

23. Which of the following is used for diagnosis of activity of disease in syphilis? ††

A. VDRL>1:64
B. VDRL > 1:16
C. VDRL > 1:8
D. VDRL > 1:2

24. Diagnosis of CNS syphilis is best done by: †

A. VDRL
B. TPHA index
C. Lymphocyte
D. Cell CT

25. Diagnosis of congenital syphilis is done by all *except:* †

A. A positive IgM EIA test
B. VDRL/RPR titre
C. TPHA
D. Biopsy

26. Match the following:

A. Benzathine pen 3 dose — a. Congenital syphilis
B. Crystalline penicillin — b. Late stage
C. Hoignes rtn — c. Early stage
D. JH rtn — d. Procaine

27. Which of the following is the drug of choice for genital warts? †

A. Podophyllin
B. Trichloroacetic acid
C. Imiquimod
D. Surgery

28. Which of the following is the drug of choice for vaginal warts?

A. Podophyllin
B. Trichloroacetic acid
C. Imiquimod
D. Surgery

29. A Gram-stained urethral smear containing should contain >=........... PMN per oil immersion field to diagnose urethritis:

A. 5
B. 10
C. 2
D. 15

30. Best therapy to cover both gonorrhoea and chlamydia is: †††

A. Azithromycin, 2 g orally as a single dose
B. Doxycycline
C. Cefixime, 400 mg orally as a single dose
D. Ceftriaxone, 250 mg intramuscular (IM) as a single dose

31. Which of the following organism is to be treated for recurrent urethritis? †††

A. Gonorrhoea
B. Chlamydia
C. Trachomoniasis
D. Herpes

Answers :

1. B	**2. AB**	**3. D**	**4. D**
5. D	**6. A**	**7. A**	**8. A**
9. C & D	**10. A & B**	**11. C**	**12. C**
13. D	**14. D**	**15. D**	**16. B**
17. B	**18. C**	**19. Ad,Bc, Cb,Da**	**20. Ad,Bc, Cb,Da**
21. A	**22. C**	**23. B**	**24. B**
25. D	**26. Ab,Ba, Cd,Dc**	**27. A**	**28. B**
29. A	**30. A**	**31. C**	

HIV*

1. Which of the following is the major core antigen in HIV? †

A. P7
B. P17
C. P24
D. P45

2. Which of the following is an envelope protein?

A. P55
B. P24
C. Gp140
D. Gp41

3. How many subtypes does HIV 1 group M have?

A. 2
B. 3
C. 11
D. 5

4. Which subtype of HIV 2 is common in India? †

A. A
B. B
C. C
D. D

5. Homosexuals usally harbour which type of HIV 2 subtype?

A. A
B. B
C. C
D. D

6. Fusion inhibitor drugs inhibit which protein? †

A. P24
B. GP120
C. P7
D. Gp41

* **Pages 113-128:** Comprehensive Textbook of Dermatology: Garg VK, Sardana K, Peepee Publishers.
Also see NACO website for HIV guidelines.

7. Which of the following are WHO stage 2 skin markers? †

A. Herpes zoster
B. Chronic herpes simplex infection
C. Persistent oral candidiasis
D. Oral hairy leukoplakia

8. Match the following:

A. WHO stage 4	a. Persistent generalized LN
B. WHO stage 3	b. Seborrheic dermatitis
C. WHO stage 1	c. Oral hairy leukoplakia
D. WHO stage 2	d. Kaposi sarcoma

9. Match the following regarding HIV testing:

A. < 350 and not on ART	a. Yearly
B. On ART (any value)	b. At 6 months
C. > 500	c. Optional
D. Anti HCV	d. At 3 months

10. Match the following:

A. NNRTI	a. Didanosine (DDL)
B. NRTI	b. Efavirenz
C. NtRTI	c. Atazanavir
D. Protease inhibitors	d. Tenofavir

11. Which of the following is not an indication initiating ART? †

A. Asymptomatic stage 1 with a CD4 < 200
B. WHO stage 3
C. WHO stage 4
D. WHO stage 2

12. ART for PEP should be started within how much time? ††

A. 1 day
B. 2 days
C. 3 days
D. 4 days

13. What therapy should you start for a mild exposure with an unknown HIV status?

A. Do nothing
B. 2 drug PEP
C. 3 drug PEP
D. Repeat HIV testing

Answers :

1. C	2. D	3. C	4. C
5. C	6. D	7. A	8. Ad,Bc,Ca,Db
9. Ad,Bb,Ca,Dc	10. Ab,Ba,Cd,Dc	11. D	12. C
13. B			

Section 3

ALLERGIC DISORDERS*

1. The most common form of drug rash is: †

A. Urticarial
B. FDE
C. SJS
D. Exanthematic

2. DRESS syndrome is caused by all *except:*

A. Sulfonamides
B. Phenobarbital
C. Valproic acid
D. Allopurinol
E. Penicillin

3. Common cause of drug induced SLE are all *except:*†

A. Hydralazine
B. Isoniazid
C. Chlorpromazine
D. Penicillamine
E. Cefuroxime

4. FDE is caused by all *except:* †

A. Penicillins
B. Tetracycline
C. Barbiturates
D. Phenolphthalein
E. Cephalosporins

5. Match the following:

A. Type I reactions	a. Rifampicin
B. Type III reactions	b. Salicylate
C. Type IV reactions	c. Neomycin sulfate
D. Type II reactions	d. Penicillin

6. P rosea like rash is caused by:

A. Arsenic
B. Tetracycline
C. Barbiturates
D. Phenolphthalein

* **Pages 132-137:** Comprehensive Textbook of Dermatology: Garg VK, Sardana K, Peepee Publishers.

7. Pemphigus vulgaris is caused by: †

A. Captopril
B. Tetracycline
C. Barbiturates
D. Phenolphthalein

8. Bullous pemphigoid like eruption is caused by:

A. Tetracycline
B. Barbiturates
C. Phenolphthalein
D. Furosemide

9. Pellagra like eruption is caused by:

A. INH
B. Tetracycline
C. Barbiturates
D. Phenolphthalein

10. Match the following:

A. Zidovudine	a Bleaching
B. Phenytoin	b. Slate grey
C. Chlorpromazine	c. Melasma
D. Chloroquine	d. Melanonychia

11. Acquired ichthyosis is caused by:

A. Clofazamine
B. Tetracycline
C. Barbiturates
D. Phenolphthalein

12. Bowen's disease is caused by:

A. Gold
B. Lead
C. Sulfonamide
D. Arsenic

13. Most common cause of acneiform eruption in India is: †

A. INH
B. Steroid
C. Phenytoin
D. Iodine

14. Match the following:

A. Type I reactions	a. Hemolysis
B. Type III reactions	b. Serum sickness
C. Type IV reactions	c. Contact dermatitis
D. Type II reactions	d. Urticaria

Answers :

1. D	**2. E**	**3. E**	**4. E**
5. Ad,Bb,Cc,Da	**6. A**	**7. A**	**8. D**
9. A	**10. Ad,Bc,Cb,Da**	**11. A**	**12. D**
13. A	**14. Ad,Bb,Cc,Da**		

ECZEMA AND DERMATITIS*

1. The most common form of contact dermatitis is:†

A. Allergic contact dermatitis
B. Irritant contact dermatitis
C. Cumulative irritant dermatitis
D. Acute irritant dermatitis

2. Which occupation has the maximum prevalence of contact dermatitis? †††

A. Drivers
B. Doctors
C. Housewife
D. Jeweller

3. Match the following: †

A. Jewellery	a. Bindi
B. Cement	b. Chromate
C. PPD	c. Hair dye
D. Paratertiary butyl phenol	d. Nickel

4. Which is the most common cause of air borne contact dermatitis in India? †

A. Parthenium
B. Insecticides
C. Dust
D. Smoke

5. Match the following:

A. Round patch	a. Asteatotic eczema
B. Sago grain	b. Pomphylox
C. HIV	c. Seborrheic dermatitis
D. Dry skin	d. Discoid eczema

6. All of the following are true about P alba *except:*†

A. Dry skin
B. Atopic
C. White non scaly macule
D. Nutritional deficiency

7. What is the most common secondary infection in atopic dermatitis due to?

A. HSV
B. MCV
C. CMV
D. S aureus

* **Pages 147-159:** Comprehensive Textbook of Dermatology: Garg VK, Sardana K, Peepee Publishers.

8. **All of the following are major features to diagnose AD *except:* †**
   A. Pruritus
   B. Family history
   C. History of asthma
   D. P alba

Answers :			
1. C	2. C	3. Ad,Bb,Cc,Da	4. A
5. Ad,Bb,Cc,Da	6. D	7. D	8. D

Section 4

COLLAGEN VASCULAR DISORDERS*

1. **Match the following: †**
   A. Anti DNA ds — a. Drug
   B. Anti RNP — b. Overlap
   C. AntiRo — c. Sjögren's
   D. Antihistone — d. Kidney

2. **Tin tack sign is seen in:**
   A. Psoriasis B. DLE
   C. Lichen planus D. Impetigo

3. **LE with lesions resembling EM are seen in:**
   A. DLE B. Rowell's syndrome
   C. SJS D. TEN

4. **Kidney involvement in SLE is best treated by: †**
   A. Steroids
   B. Steroids + Azathioprine
   C. Steroids + Cyclophosphamide
   D. Chloroquine

5. **Which of the following is the drug preferred for skin rash of LE? †**
   A. Aspirin B. Chloroquine
   C. Retinoids D. Steroids

6. **Match the following: †**
   A. Tendon friction rubs — a. CREST
   B. U1-RNP positive — b. Overlap
   C. Digital pitted scars — c. Minor criterian
   D. Pulmonary hypertension — d. Diffuse PSS

7. **Which of the following is not used for Raynaud phenomenon?**
   A. Nifedipine
   B. Verapamil hydrochloride
   C. Losartan potassium
   D. D penicillamine

8. **All are used for pulmonary hypertension *except:***
   A. Epoprostenol
   B. Iloprost
   C. Steroids
   D. Verapamil

9. **All are used for kidney involvement *except:***
   A. Captopril
   B. Enalapril malate
   C. Kidney dialysis
   D. Etanercept

10. **All are antifibrotics *except:***
    A. D-penicillamine B. Colchicine
    C. Nifedipine D. Relaxin

11. **All are causes of occupational scleroderma *except:***
    A. Vinyl chloride B. Malathion/Parathion
    C. Epoxy resins D. Lead

12. **All of the following are seen in dermatomyosistis *except:* †**
    A. Heliotrope erythema
    B. Periungual telangiectasias
    C. Shawl sign
    D. Oral ulcers

13. **Match the following:**
    A. Anti SRP — a. PSS
    B. Anti Jo 1 — b. Mechanics hand
    C. Anti Ku — c. LE
    D. Anti PM–Scl antibody — d. CVS

Answers :			
1. Ad,Bb,Cc,Da	2. B	3. B	4. C
5. B	6. Ad,Bb,Cc,Da	7. D	8. D
9. D	10. C	11. D	12. D
13. Ad,Bb,Cc,Da			

* **Pages 164-177:** Comprehensive Textbook of Dermatology: Garg VK, Sardana K, Peepee Publishers.

VESICULOBULLOUS DISORDERS*

1. Match the following: †

A. Suprabasal — a. Impetigo
B. Tense bulla — b. Bullous pemphigoid
C. Subepidermal — c. PCT
D. Suborneal — d. Pemphigus vulgaris

2. Match the following:

A. Dsg 3 — a. Iga pemphigus
B. Collagen 7 — b. EB dystrohica
C. BPAg 1 — c. BP
D. Desmocollins 1 and 2 — d. Pemphigus vulgaris

3. All are seen in pemphigus vulgaris *except:* †

A. Oral involvement B. Flaccid bulla
C. Nikolsky sign D. Itch

4. All are seen in pemphigus vulgaris *except:*

A. Row of tombstones B. Fish-net
C. IgG D. IgA

5. Drug induced pemphigus is usually: †

A. P. vulgaris B. P foliaceous
C. IgA pemphigus D. Endemic type

6. Black fly causes:

A. P. vulgaris
B. P foliaceous
C. IgA pemphigus
D. Endemic type of pemphigus foliacious

7. Best prognosis is seen in:

A. P. vulgaris B. Neonatal type
C. IgA pemphigus D. Endemic type

8. All are seen in bullous pemphigoid *except:* †

A. Tense B. Itchy
C. Urticaria D. Self limiting

9. Scarring is seen in:

A. Pemphigus
B. Cicatricial pemphigoid
C. DH
D. Urticaria

10. Which of the following is not seen in herpes gestationis? †

A. Tense bulla B. Periumbilical
C. C3 D. HSV2

11. A patient comes with chronic itchy papulovesicle on the extensors which of the following is not true? †

A. Aggravated by wheat
B. Dapsone helps
C. IgA granular
D. Subcorneal split

12. Ring of pearl is seen in: ††

A. Pemphigus B. Pemphigoid
C. CBDC D. IgA pemphigus

13. Mitten hands is seen in:

A. EB simplex B. EB junctionalis
C. EB dystrophica D. DH

14. Match the following:

A. Intercellular IgG — a. Bullous pemphigoid
B. C3 — b. Herpes gestationis
C. IgA1 — c. DH
D. Linear IgG — d. Pemphigus vulgaris

Answers :

1. Ad, Bb, Cc, Da	2. Ad, Bb, Cc, Da	3. D	4. D
5. B	6. D	7. B	8. D
9. B	10. D	11. D	12. C
13. C	14. Ad, Bb, Cc, Da		

Section 5

PAPULOSQUAMOUS DISORDERS**

1. Match the following: †

A. Normal cell cycle time — a. 53 days
B. Psoriasis — b. 7 days
C. Psoriatic turnover time — c. 36 hours
D. Cell turnover time — d. 311 hours

2. Which of the following is a strong risk factor for plaque psoriasis?

A. HLA CW6 B. HLA B27
C. HLA B3 D. HLA C6

3. Papulosquamous lesions preceded by sore throat is seen in: †

A. Plaque psoriasis
B. Guttate type
C. Pustular type
D. Erythroderma

* **Page 183:** Extremely Important – MUST READ—Comprehensive Textbook of Dermatology: Garg VK, Sardana K, Peepee Publishers.
** **MUST READ–Pages 207-225:** Comprehensive Textbook of Dermatology: Garg VK, Sardana K, Peepee Publishers.

4. All of the following are form of pustular psoriasis *except:* †

A. Von Zumbusch's
B. Palm and sole
C. Acrodermatitis erythroderma
D. Impetigo herpetiforms

5. Which of the following is the most *characteristic form* of nail psoriasis? ††

A. Pitting
B. Oildrop sign
C. Subungual hyperkeratosis
D. Onycholysis

6. Pityriasis (tinea) amiantacea is another name for psoriasis of the:

A. Palm B. Sole
C. Nail D. Scalp

7. The most common form of psoriatic arthritis is: †

A. Asymmetrical oligoarthritis
B. RA like
C. Mutilans
D. Distal IP joint

8. All are true in psoriasis *except:* †

A. Parakeratosis
B. Munro's microabscess
C. Spongiform pustules
D. Hypergranulosis

9. Match the following:

A. Plaque a. Methotrexate
B. Pustular b. Steroid
C. Impetigo herpetiformis c. Acitretin
D. Erythroderma d. PUVA

10. Which of the following is a topical retinoid used in psoriasis?

A. Tretinoin B. Tazarotene
C. Methotrexate D. Steroid

11. Short contact therapy is used for:

A. Steroid B. Tar
C. Anthralin D. Tacrolimus

12. Match the following: †

A. Etanercept a. Lymphocyte
B. Efalizumab b. LFA-3
C. Alefacept c. CD11a
D. Methotrexate d. TNF-alpha

13. Island of sparing is classically seen in: †

A. PRP B. P rosea
C. Erythroderma D. Psoriasis

14. Classic histology of PRP shows:

A. Hypergranulosis
B. Dilation of vessels
C. BMZ zone loss
D. Checkerboard pattern

15. All are true about seborrheic dermatitis *except:*

A. Aggravate in summer
B. Seen in Parkinson's disease
C. Antifungal help
D. Recurs

16. Pityriasis rosea is characterized by all *except:* †

A. Christmas tree pattern B. Herald patch
C. Viral infection D. Antifungal help

17. Most likely cause of P rosea is: †

A. HHV-2 B. HHV-5
C. HHV-6 D. HHV-7

18. All of the following don't cause medication-induced P rosae *except:*

A. Captopril B. Isotretinoin
C. Terbinafine D. Ivermectin

19. Graham Little Piccardi syndrome is characterized by all *except:*

A. Lichen planus
B. Cicatricial alopecia of axilla
C. Non-cicatricial alopecia on axillary
D. Follicular lesions

20. Reticular lesions are seen in: †

A. Mucosa B. Scalp
C. Axilla D. Nail

21. All are seen in the nail of LP *except:* †

A. Distal splitting B. Onychogryposis
C. Pterygium D. Pup tent sign

22. DIF in LP shows:

A. IgM B. IgG
C. IgA D. C3

Answers :

1. Ad, Bc, Cb, Da	2. A	3. B	4. C
5. B	6. D	7. A	8. D
9. Ad, Bc, Cb, Da	10. B	11. C	12. Ad, Bc, Cb, Da
13. A	14. D	15. A	16. D
17. D	18. A	19. B	20. A
21. B	22. A		

Section 6

PHOTO DERMATOLOGY*

1. **Match the following:**

A. UVA	a. Animals
B. Burns	b. UVB
C. UVA1	c. 340-400
D. UVC	d. Majority of UVR

2. **In India the skin type is:**
   A. Type 1 B. Type 2
   C. Type 3 D. Type 4

3. **Meirowsky phenomenon is: †**
   A. Immediate tanning
   B. Sunburn
   C. Delayed tanning
   D. Cancer causing radiation

4. **Photoageing is all *except:***
   A. Fibroelastolytic papulosis
   B. Cutis rhomboidalis nuchae
   C. Favre-Racouchit syndrome
   D. Milia

5. **Most common form of PMLE is:**
   A. Papular form B. Vesicle
   C. Bulla D. Nodule

6. **Pocklike scarring is seen in:**
   A. PMLE
   B. Actinic prurigo
   C. Hydroa vacciniforme
   D. Urticaria

Answers :

1. Ad, Bb, Cc, Da	2. D	3. A	4. D
5. A	6. C		

METABOLIC DISORDERS *

1. **Which of the following is diagnostic of macular amyloidosis?**
   A. Rippled pigmentation B. Nodules
   C. Vesicles D. Bulla

2. **Which type of amyloid is seen in nodular amyloidosis? †**
   A. AL B. AA
   C. AK D. AM

3. **Secondary cutaneous amyloidosis is characterized by:**
   A. AL B. AA
   C. AK D. AM

4. **Macroglossia, purpura, periorbital (Raccoon sign) are seen with deposition of:**
   A. AL B. AA
   C. AK D. Am

5. **Severe photosensitivity with blistering, scarring and mutilation of the exposed parts, and red urine and teeth is seen:**
   A. PCT
   B. Gunther's diseases
   C. Erythrohepatic protoporphyria
   D. Variegate porphyria

6. **Crusted vesicles, leading to pitted scars are seen all *except*: †**
   A. PCT
   B. Gunther's diseases
   C. Erythrohepatic protoporphyria
   D. Variegate porphyria

7. **An male alcoholic comes with blisters, erosions and milia form on the exposed parts of the face and on the backs of the hands, what is it?**
   A. PCT
   B. Gunther's diseases
   C. Erythrohepatic protoporphyria
   D. Variegate porphyria

8. **A fair skin patient comes with atopic eczema and has mental retardation what is the most likely diagnosis?**

* **Pages 230-238 :** Comprehensive Textbook of Dermatology: Garg VK, Sardana K, Peepee Publishers.

A. Wiskott-Aldrich phenomenon
B. Ataxia telangiectasia
C. Phenylketonuria
D. Scurvy

9. Match the following:

A. Alkaptonuria — a. Marfanoid habitus
B. Keratoderma — b. Richner hanhart
C. Pellagra — c. Dark urine
D. Homocystinuria — d. Hartnup disease

Answers :

1. A	**2. A**	**3. C**	**4. A**
5. B	**6. C**	**7. A**	**8. C**
9. Ac,Bb,Cd,Da			

GENODERMATOSES*

1. Match the following in NF 1: †

A. Most common skin tumor — a. 17
B. Most common systemic tumor — b. Optic nerve gliomas
C. Pigmentation in axilla — c. Neurofibroma
D. Chromosome — d. Crowe's sign

2. Bourneville's disease: †

A. Tuberous sclerosis
B. NF
C. Ataxia telangiectasia
D. Marfan's disease

3. Which of the following are major features of tuberous sclerosis:

A. Shagreen patch
B. Cortical tuber
C. Hypomelanotic macules
D. Gingival fibromas

4. Which of the following is the earliest systemic tumor in tuberous sclerosis? †

A. Subependymal giant cell astrocytoma
B. Cardiac rhabdomyoma
C. Lymphangiomyomatosis
D. Renal angiomyolipoma

5. Match the following TSC:

A. Koenens tumor — a. 9
B. Shagreen patch — b. Back
C. Gardner's syndrome — c. Mucosal papillomas
D. Chromosome — d. Nail

6. Match the following:

A. Bloom's syndrome — a. BCC
B. Cockayne syndrome — b. XL dominant
C. Incontinentia pigmenti — c. Mickey mouse faces
D. Xeroderma pigmentosa — d. Butterfly area

7. Match the following:

A. Cutaneous mosaicism — a. Unna Thost syndrome
B. Goltz syndrome — b. PJ syndrome
C. Intestinal polyps — c. Dermal hyoplasia
D. Keratoderma — d. Hypomelanosis of Ito

8. A patient presents with scaly, waxy, greasy papules in the seborrheic areas. The oral mucosa shows palatal papules: †

A. Seborrheic dermatitis
B. LP
C. Hailey-Hailey disease
D. Darier's disease

9. Corps ronds and grains are seen in: †

A. Seborrheic dermatitis
B. LP
C. Hailey-Hailey disease
D. Darier's disease

10. Match the following:

A. Non-bullous congenital ichthyosiform erythroderma — a. Filaggrin
B. Lamellar ichthyosis — b. Lamellar bodies
C. Recessive X-linked ichthyosis — c. Transglutaminase
D. Ichthyosis vulgaris — d. Steroid sulfatase

Answers :

1. Ac,Bb,Cd,Da	**2. A**	**3. A, B**	**4. B**
5. Ad,Bb,Cc,Da	**6. Ad,Bc,Cb,Da**	**7. Ad,Bc,Cb,Da**	**8. D**
9. D	**10. Ab, Bc,Cd,Da**		

Page 245: Comprehensive Textbook of Dermatology: Garg VK, Sardana K, Peepee Publishers.

PIGMENTARY DISORDERS*

1. Which of the following is the red pigment forming cell?

A. Eumelanins
B. Phaeomelanins
C. Seomelanin
D. Tyrosine

2. Which of the following is blanchable and present at birth? †

A. Nevus depigmentosus
B. Nevus anemicus
C. Piebaldism
D. Vitiligo

3. Which of the following involves the midline?

A. Nevus depigmentosus B. Nevus anemicus
C. Piebaldism D. Vitiligo

4. Which of the following conditions does not involve the melanocytes but is still white at birth? †

A. Woronoff ring
B. Nevus depigmentosus
C. Nevus anemicus
D. Piebaldism

5. Piebaldism hypertelorism and deafness is seen in:

A. Nevus depigmentosus
B. Nevus anemicus
C. Woolf syndrome
D. Waardenburg's syndrome

6. Which form of vitiligo remain stable for life?

A. Classical B. Acrofacial
C. Segmental D. Generalised

7. For localized disease vitiligo in children all are given *except:* †

A. NB UVB B. Tacrolimus
C. Top steroid D. Syst steroid

8. Silver-gray hair, recurrent infection, seizures and pancytopenia is seen in:

A. Cross syndrome
B. Griscelli syndrome
C. Hermansky-Pudlak
D. Chediak-Higashi

9. Bleeding diathesis is classically seen in:

A. Cross syndrome
B. Griscelli syndrome
C. Hermansky-Pudlak
D. Chediak-Higashi

10. All are true about P alba *except:*

A. Erythema
B. Scale
C. Eczematous dermatosis
D. PUVA should be given

11. In which of the following are melanocytes increased? †

A. Lentigines B. Freckles
C. Ochronosis D. Alkaptonuria

12. In which syndrome are multiple lentigines associated with gastrointestinal polyposis, alopecia and nail abnormalities? †

A. Cronkhite-Canada syndrome
B. Peutz-Jeghers syndrome
C. N spilius
D. Name syndrome

13. All of the following are blue in colour *except:*

A. N of ota B. N of ito
C. Melasma D. Hori nevus

14. Match the following conditions:

A. Argyria	a. Pressure points
B. Chrysoderma	b. Red
C. Clofazimine	c. Gold
D. Hydroxyurea	d. Silver

15. Match the following:

A. Tyrosinase inhibitors	a. Azelaic acid
B. Antioxidants	b. Ascorbic acid
C. Melanogenesis inhibitors	c. Retinoic acid
D. Exfoliants	d. Glycolic acid

16. Match the following conditions with CALM:

A. McCune-Albright	a. Polyostotic fibrous dysplasia
B. Fanconi's anemia	b. Pulmonary stenosis
C. Watson syndrome	c. Pancytopenia
D. Russell-Sliver syndrome	d. Short stature

* **Page 256:** Comprehensive Textbook of Dermatology: Garg VK, Sardana K, Peepee Publishers.

17. Match the following conditions:

A. Riehl's melanosis	a. PPD
B. Berloque dermatitis	b. Eau de cologne
C. Erythema dyschromicum perstans	c. Gum line
D. Bismuth	d. Tar derivatives

Answers :

1. B	2. B	3. C	4. C
5. D	6. C	7. D	8. D
9. C	10. D	11. A	12. D
13. C	14. Ad,Bc,Cb,Da	15. Aa,Bb,Cc,Dd	
16. Aa,Bc,Cb,Dd	17. Ad,Bb,Ca,Dc		

Section 7

TUMORS OF THE SKIN*

1. Sign of Leser-Trélat is seen with:†

A. Seborrheic keratosis
B. Dysplastic nevus syndrome
C. Myelosis leukemia
D. Pseudolymphoma of spiegler

2. Chronic nodule with a central crater filled with horny, hyperkeratotic material is seen in:

A. Warty dyskeratoma
B. Keratoacanthoma
C. Arsenical keratosis
D. Kraurosis vulvae

3. All are sebaceous tumors *except:*

A. Milia
B. Nevus sebaceous
C. Adenoma sebaceum
D. Sebaceous hyperplasia

4. A nevus with a depigmented area surrounding it is called:

A. Junctional nevi B. Intradermal nevi
C. Sutton's nevus D. Lentigo

5. Spontaneously resolution is seen in:

A. Hemangioma
B. PWS
C. Salmon patch
D. Parkes Weber syndrome

6. Consumption coagulopathy is seen in: †

A. Kasabach-Merritt syndrome
B. Cherry hemangiomas
C. Fabry disease
D. Gorham syndrome

7. Match the following conditions:

A. Disappearing bones	a. Phaces syndrome
B. Enchondromas	b. Maffucci syndrome
C. Stridor	c. Cobb syndrome
D. Neurologic manifestations	d. Gorham's disease

Answers :

1. A	2. B	3. A,C	4. C
5. A	6. A	7. Ad,Bb,Ca,Dc	

Section 8

DISORDERS OF THE MUCOSA AND HAIR**

1. Sutton's disease is basically another name for: †

A. Hand-foot-mouth disease
B. Aphthous stomatitis
C. Ludwig's angina
D. Trench mouth

2. Cayenne pepper appearance: †

A. Erythroplasia of queyrat
B. Zoon's balanitis
C. Neurodermatitis
D. Erythrasma

3. Which of the following is seen in infants?

A. Lanugo B. Vellus
C. Terminal hair D. Kenogen

4. Eflornithine hydrochloride is a new drug for: †

A. Hypertrichois B. Melasma
C. Multiple sclerosis D. Poems syndrome

5. Non-scarring alopecia is seen in all *except:* †

A. Telogen effluvium
B. Anagen effluvium
C. Loose anagen syndrome
D. Aplasia cutis congenital

* **Page 273:** Comprehensive Textbook of Dermatology: Garg VK, Sardana K, Peepee Publishers.

** **Page 295:** MUST READ–Disorders of Hairs and Nails (306-22) Comprehensive Textbook of Dermatology: Garg VK, Sardana K, Peepee Publishers.

6. **Scarring alopecia is seen in all *except*: †**
   A. Alopecia areata
   B. Pseudopelade of brocq
   C. Graham-Little syndrome
   D. D.L.E.

7. **Christmas tree pattern is seen in:**
   A. Female AGA　B. A male AGA
   C. AA　D. Telogen effluvium

8. **DOC in males with MAGA:†**
   A. Minoxidil 5%　B. Afinasteride 1 mg
   C. Minoxidil 2%　D. Dutasteride

9. **The average time interval between the stress and hair loss in telogen effluvium: ††**
   A. 2 m　B. 3 m
   C. 1 m　D. 4 m

10. **Lymphocytic scarring alopecia is seen in all *except*:**
    A. Central centrifugal cicatricial alopecia (CCCA)
    B. Discoid lupus
    C. Lichen planopilaris (LPP)
    D. Folliculitis decalvans

11. **Match the following conditions:**

A. Trichoschisis	a. Wooly hair
B. Trichorrhexis invaginata	b. Bamboo hair
C. No hair fragility	c. Trichorrhexis nodosa
D. Menke's syndrome	d. Transverse split

12. **Pits in the nail are seen in all *except*: †**
    A. Psoriasis　B. Alopecia areata
    C. Nail biting　D. Lichen planus

13. **Onychocryptosis is another name for:**
    A. Ingrowing toe nail
    B. Subungual hematoma
    C. Racket nail
    D. Paronychia

14. **Inflammation of the proximal nail fold is seen in:**
    A. Ingrowing toe nail
    B. Subungual hematoma
    C. Racket nail
    D. Paronychia

15. **Inverted fir tree configuration is seen in:**
    A. Ingrowing toe nail
    B. Subungual hematoma
    C. Racket nail
    D. Habit-tic deformity

16. **Trachyonychia is seen in all *except:***
    A. Lichen planus　B. Psoriasis
    C. Alopecia areata　D. Paronychia

17. **Most characteristic nail defect in psoriasis is: †**
    A. Onycholyis
    B. Pitting
    C. Oil drop sign
    D. Subungual hyperkeratosis

18. **Geometric pitting is seen in: ††**
    A. Lichen planus　B. Psoriasis
    C. Alopecia areata　D. Paronychia

19. **Pterygium is seen in all *except:* ††**
    A. Lichen planus　B. Radiotherapy
    C. Trauma　D. Psoriasis

20. **V-shaped distal notching is seen in:**
    A. LP　B. Psoriasis
    C. Darier's disease　D. Tine unguim

21. **Match the following conditions:**

A. Pseudoleukonychia	a. CRF
B. Terry's nail	b. Cirrhosis
C. Half-and-half	c. Pseudomonas
D. Green nails	d. Onychomycosis

22. **Half-and-half nail is because of: †**
    A. Vascular compromise
    B. Increased melanin deposition
    C. Keratin defect
    D. All of the above

Answers :

1. B	2. B	3. A	4. A
5. D	6. A	7. A	8. A
9. B	10. D	11. Ad, Bb, Ca, Dc	12. D
13. A	14. D	15. D	16. D
17. C	18. C	19. D	20. C
21. Ad, Bb, Ca, Dc	22. D		

DISORDERS OF APPENDAGEAL GLANDS*

1. **Which of the following is a self-induced acne? †**
   A. Acne excoriee des jeunes files
   B. Steroid acne
   C. Halogen acne
   D. Occupational acne

2. **Which of the following is classically monomorphic? †**
   A. Acne excoriee des jeunes files
   B. Steroid acne
   C. Halogen acne
   D. Occupational acne

3. **Summer sunlight induced acne is also called:**
   A. Acne excoriee des jeunes files
   B. Acne aestivalis
   C. Halogen acne
   D. Occupational acne

4. **Which of the following is mainly comedolytic?**
   A. Retinoids B. Benzoyl peroxide
   C. Clindamycin D. Azelaic acid

5. **Drug of choice in an *unmarried female* with acne is: †**
   A. Isotretinoin B. Minocycline
   C. Azithromycin D. Septran

6. **A female with acne not responding to isotretinoin is most likely suffering from: ††**
   A. PCOS B. Acne conglobata
   C. Steroid acne D. Acne pustulosa

7. **Which of the following is a newer drug for hyperhidrosis?**
   A. Potassium permanganate soaks
   B. Glutaraldehyde
   C. 20% aluminium chloride hexahydrate
   D. BTX-A

8. **A child come with high grade fever, sweating and small white papules on the trunk the most likely cause is: †**
   A. Miliaria crystallina B. Miliaria rubra
   C. Miliaria profunda D. Milia

9. **Itchy papules on the axillae breasts and vulva is seen in: †**
   A. Miliaria
   B. Tinea
   C. Fox Fordyce's disease
   D. Fordyce's spots

Answers :

1. A	2. B	3. B	4. A	5. A
6. C	7. D	8. A	9. C	

Section 9

DERMATOLOGICAL SIGNS OF INTERNAL DISEASE**

1. **Hyperextensibility, hypermobility, skin fragility and "fish-mouth" scars, are seen in:**
   A. Pseudoxanthoma elasticum
   B. Ehlers-Danlos syndrome
   C. Sarcoidosis
   D. Cutis laxa

2. **Which of the following is a vasculitis:**
   A. Pyoderma gangrenosum
   B. Sarcoidosis
   C. Cutis laxa
   D. L. planus

3. **All are features of hyperthyroidism *except:***
   A. Pretibial myxedema
   B. Thyroid acropachy
   C. Exophthalmos
   D. Acne

4. **All of the following are associated with Fitz Curths criteria *except:* †**
   A. Bazex's syndrome
   B. Carcinoid syndrome
   C. Erythema gyratum repens
   D. Pityriasis rotunda

5. **Match the following conditions:**
   A. Vitamin B_{12} a. Edema
   B. Vitamin C b. Follicular keratosis

---

* **Pages 334-338:** Comprehensive Textbook of Dermatology: Garg VK, Sardana K, Peepee Publishers.

** **Page 344:** Comprehensive Textbook of Dermatology: Garg VK, Sardana K, Peepee Publishers.

C. Kwashiorkor	c. Diarrhoea and dementia
D. Niacin	d. Hyperpigmentation

6. In which nutritional deficiency are the finger flexural creases and the palms affected showing characteristic flat, grayish, bullous lesions surrounded by red-brown erythema? †

A. Vitamin A
B. Zn
C. Vitamin B
D. Vitamin D

7. Match the following conditions:

A. Rifoflavin	a. Butterfly area
B. Haemochromatosis	b. Cirrhosis
C. Vitamin A	c. Phrynoderma
D. Niacin	d. Glossitis

Answers :

1. B	2. A	3. D	4. D
5. Ad,Bb,Ca,Dc	6. B	7. Ad,Bb,Cc,Da	

PSYCHOCUTANEOUS DISORDERS*

1. Ekbom's disease is also known as: †

A. Delusions of body image
B. Delusions of parasitosis
C. Syphilophobia
D. Compulsive hand washing

2. All of the following have visible cutaneous features *except:*

A. Dermatitis artefacta
B. Witchcraft syndrome
C. Dermatological pathomimicry
D. Munchausen's syndrome

3. Which of the following is a body image disorder?

A. Trichotillomania
B. Acne excoriée
C. Onychotillomania
D. Psychogenic purpuras

4. Friar tuck appearance is seen in: †

A. Dermatitis artefacta
B. Witchcraft syndrome
C. Dermatological pathomimicry
D. Trichotillomania

5. Gardner-Diamond syndrome refers to:

A. Trichotillomania
B. Acne excoriée
C. Onychotillomania
D. Psychogenic purpuras

Answers :

1. B	2. D	3. B	4. D
5. D			

MISCELLANEOUS INFILTRATIVE DISORDERS*

1. Which of the following mimic's cellulites but pathologically shows only eosinophils?

A. Wells' syndrome
B. Hypereosinophilic syndrome
C. Churg-Strauss syndrome
D. Kimura disease

2. Which of the following is the most common cause of eosinophilic infiltration?

A. Hypereosinophilic syndrome
B. Churg-Strauss syndrome
C. Kimura disease
D. Drug eruption

3. Which of the following figurate erythema is characterized by a trailing scale?

A. Erythema annulare centrifugum
B. Erythema chronicum migrans
C. Erythema marginatum
D. Erythema gyratum repens

4. Which of the following figurate erythema is seen in rheumatic fever?

A. Erythema annulare centrifugum
B. Erythema chronicum migrans
C. Erythema marginatum
D. Erythema gyratum repens

5. Match the following conditions:

A. Epithelioid granulomas	a. Sarcoidosis
B. Foreign-body granulomas	b. Silica
C. Necrobiotic annulare	c. Granuloma
D. Perifollicular granuloma	d. Lichen scrofulosorum

6. Darier's sign is seen: ††

A. Erythema annulare centrifugum

* **Pages 358 and 386-392:** Comprehensive Textbook of Dermatology: Garg VK, Sardana K, Peepee Publishers.

B. Erythema chronicum migrans
C. Urticaria pigmentosa
D. Angioedema

7. A child comes with severe seborrheic rash, with crusted papular lesions, erosions, what is the most likely diagnosis? †
A. Juvenile xanthogranuloma
B. Generalized eruptive histiocytosis
C. Xanthoma disseminatum
D. Langerhans cell histiocytosis

8. All are metastatic calcification *except:*
A. Hematomas
B. Hyperparathyroidism
C. Pseudohypoparathyroidism
D. Chronic renal failure

9. A condition affecting women with white patches circling the vulva and anus take on an hourglass shape is seen in: †
A. Vitiligo
B. Lichen planus
C. Balanitis xerotica obliterans
D. Lichen sclerosus

10. Match the following conditions:

A. Madelung disease	a. Lipomatosis
B. Septal, panniculitis	b. Erythema nodosum
C. Plucked chicken	c. Pseudoxanthoma elasticum
D. Peau d'orange	d. Pretibial myxedema

Answers :

1. A	**2. D**	**3. A**	**4. C**
5. Aa,Bb,Cc,Dd	**6. C**	**7. D**	**8. A**
9. D	**10. Aa,Bb,Cc,Dd**		

Section 10

THERAPY*

1. FTU (Finger tip unit) is equal to:
A. 0.5 gm B. 1 gm
C. 2 gm D. 3 gm

2. Acne preparations are:
A. Gel B. Ointment
C. Cream D. Lotion

3. Match the following steroids with the potency: ††

A. Superpotency	a. Methyprednisolone cream
B. Potent	b. Mometasone furoate
C. Moderate potent	c. Clobetasol propionate
D. Mild	d. Prednicarbate cream

4. All of the following retinoids are used in acne *except:* †
A. Tretinoin B. Adapalene
C. Isotretinoin D. Tazarotene

5. The safest topical agent for acne is:
A. Sulphur-2-10% B. Tretinoin
C. Adapalene D. Azelaic acid

6. All of the following are known to stain the skin in psoriasis *except:*
A. Coal tar B. Dithranol
C. Tazarotene D. Calcipotriene

7. Which of the following antifungal is an allylamine? †
A. Terbinafine B. Nystatin
C. Amorolfine D. Undecylenic acid

8. Keratoplastic agents is one of the following:
A. Salicylic acid (1% to 2%)
B. Sulfur (4% to 10%)
C. Urea
D. Salicylic acid (2% to 4%)

9. Which of the following is given for both dermatophyte and candida? ††
A. Nystatin B. Amphotericin B
C. Clotrimazole D. Terbinafine

10. All are non-sedating antihistamines, *except:*
A. Acrivastine B. Loratadine
C. Fexofenadine D. Cyproheptadine

11. TPMT testing is done for:
A. Azathioprine B. Methotrexate
C. Cyclophosphamide D. Cyclosporine

* **Pages 398-426:** Comprehensive Textbook of Dermatology: Garg VK, Sardana K, Peepee Publishers.

12. All are used for acne *except:* †

A. Isotretinoin
B. Oral contraceptives
C. Minocycline
D. Fucidin

13. Thalidomide is given in all *except:* ††

A. Aphthous ulceration
B. Codular prurigo
C. Erythema nodosum leprosum
D. Sweet's syndrome

14. Match the following biological agents:

A. Alefacept	a. Banned
B. Etanercept	b. TNF alpha
C. Infliximab	c. Fusion protein
D. Efalizumab	d. IV

15. The safest peel for Indian skin is: †

A. Lactic acid
B. Glycolic acid
C. Pyruvic acid
D. Salicylic acid

16. Self neutralising peel is: †

A. Lactic acid
B. Glycolic acid
C. Pyruvic acid
D. Salicylic acid

17. Best laser for hair removal in Indian skin is:

A. IPL B. Diode
C. NdYAG D. LED

18. Laser of choice for pigmented skin is:

A. IPL B. Diode
C. NdYAG D. LED

Answers :

1. A	**2. A**	**3. Ac,Bb,Cd,Da**	**4. D**
5. A	**6. D**	**7. A**	**8. A**
9. C	**10. D**	**11. A**	**12. D**
13. D	**14. Ac,Bb,Cd,Da**	**15. D**	**16. D**
17. C	**18. C**		

Part III

Exam Based MCQs

A Summary of Basic and Common MCQs Asked in Exams: Section-wise.
This section must be read before any PG exam. Our analysis of last 2 years have shown that maximum Q come from this section.

How to use	*Chapters that are important*	*Exams relevant*
This is topic-wise compilation of ACTUAL MCQs of exams † Important MCQs wrongly answered in guide books †† Most Important MCQs ††† Extremely Important MCQs	Introduction Infections Infestations STD HIV Allergic diseases Bullous disorders Papulosquamous Pigmented disorders Therapy	AIPG AIIMS PGI UPSC Delhi PG State Exams

Section 1

INTRODUCTION OF SKIN DISEASES

1. **Tzanck cell is a: †**
   A. Lymphocyte
   B. Monocyte
   C. Neutrophil
   D. Keratinocyte
   E. Eosinophil

2. **In which of the following is the Wood's light colour green?**
   A. Urine examination in porphyria
   B. Hair in T. capitis
   C. P versicolor
   D. All of the above

3. **Herald patch is the first feature of:**
   A. Pityriasis rosea B. Pemphigus
   C. Psoriasis D. Leprosy

4. **Which of the following is a self-limiting condition?**
   A. Scabies
   B. Impetigo contagiosa
   C. Molluscum contagiosa
   D. Psoriasis

5. **Skin doubling time is: ††**
   A. 1 week B. 2 weeks
   C. 4 weeks D. 8 weeks

6. **Diagnostic method of choice in contact dermatitis is:**
   A. Patch test B. Tzanck test
   C. Skin biopsy D. Intradermal test

7. **A pinkish red fluorescence of urine with Wood's lamp is seen in:**
   A. Lead poisoning
   B. Porphyria cutanea tarda
   C. Erythromelagia
   D. Acrocyanosis

8. **The time required for a cell of S basale to reach the S corneum is:**
   A. 4 days B. 12 days
   C. 28 days D. 35 days

9. **Which laser is selectively absorbed by water?**
   A. Argon B. CO_2
   C. Ruby D. YAG

10. **Which of the following is burrow's solution?**
    A. Aluminium subacetate
    B. Silvernitrate
    C. Potassium permagnate
    D. Sodium thiosulfate

11. **The topical antibiotic that has a structural analogy to steroid is:**
    A. Gentian violet B. Gentamicin
    C. Fucidin D. Acriflavine

12. **Which of the following is the most specific marker for Langerhan's cells? ††**
    A. CD 1a B. S 100
    C. CD 100 D. Peanut agglutinin

13. **Patch test is read after: ††**
    A. 2 hours B. 2 days
    C. 4 days D. 2 months

14. **Atopic dermatitis can be best diagnosed by:**
    A. Clinical evaluation B. Patch test
    C. IgE level D. Biopsy

15. **Exclamation mark hairs are seen in:**
    A. Syphilis B. Alopecia areata
    C. Psoriasis D. Dermatophytosis

16. **Growth phase of hair is:**
    A. Anagen B. Metagen
    C. Telogen D. None

17. **Munro micro abscess is seen in:**
    A. Dermal tissue B. Stratum basale
    C. Stratum corneum D. Stratum malpighi

18. **Melanocytes are present in:**
    A. Stratum corneum
    B. Stratum basale
    C. Stratum granulosum
    D. Dermal tissue

19. **Basal cell degeneration seen in:**
    A. Lichen planus B. Psoriasis
    C. Pemphigus D. EM

20. Which of the following is an abnormality of eccrine gland?

A. Milia
B. Syringoma
C. Miliaria
D. Trichoepithelioma

21. Which of the following can be depressed?

A. Sec. syphilis
B. Dermatitis herpetiformis
C. Psoriasis
D. Morphoea
E. Plaque

22. The test likely to help in diagnosis of a patient who presents with an itchy annular plaque on the face is:

A. Gram's stain
B. Potassium hydroxide mount
C. Tissue smear
D. Wood's lamp examination

23. Which layer of epidermis is underdeveloped in the VLBW infants in the initial 7 days?

A. Stratum germinativum
B. Stratum granulosum
C. Stratum lucidum
D. Stratum corneum

24. Nikolsky sign is positive in all *except:*

A. Pemphigus
B. Bullous pemphigoid
C. Toxic epidermonecrolysis
D. Staphylococcal scalded skin syndrome

25. Normal turnover time for epidermis is: †††

A. 2 weeks
B. 4 weeks
C. 6 weeks
D. 8 weeks

26. Isomorphic response is seen in all *except*:

A. DLE
B. Lichen planus
C. Psoriasis
D. Pemphigus

27. One melanocyte supplies:

A. 10 keratinocytes
B. 36 keratinocytes
C. 45 keratinocytes
D. 20 keratinocytes

28. Huxley's and Henley's layer is a part of:

A. Hair
B. Nail
C. Skin
D. Sweat gland

29. The turnover time of the epidermis is: ††

A. 7 days
B. 14 days
C. 21 days
D. 56 days

30. Berkeley's membrane is seen in:

A. Pemphigus
B. Psoriasis
C. Pityriasis rosea
D. Pemphigoid

31. Stratum lucidum is seen in:

A. Hair and nails
B. Palms and soles
C. Normal epidermis
D. Scalp

32. Birbeck granules are part of:

A. Langerhans cells
B. Keratinocytes
C. Melanocytes
D. Merkel cells

Answers :

1. D	2. B,C	3. A	4. C
5. C	6. A	7. B	8. C
9. B	10. A	11. C	12. D
13. C	14. A	15. B	16. A
17. C	18. B	19. A	20. B,C
21. D,E	22. B	23. D	24. B
25. D	26. D	27. B	28. A
29. D	30. B	31. B	32. A

Section 2

FUNGAL INFECTION

1. The most common cause of dermatophytosis is:

A. Malassezia furfur
B. Candida
C. Trichophyton rubrum
D. Trichophyton mentagrophyte

2. Which of the following mimics white psoriasis?

A. Tinea capitis
B. Tinea corporis
C. Tinea pedis
D. T mannum
E. All of the above

3. Treatment of tinea versicolor is all *except*:

A. Clotrimazole
B. Sytemic terbinafine
C. Selenium sulphide
D. Griseofulvin
E. Top terbinafine

4. A cystic, boggy swelling over scalp with easily pluckable hair the drug of choice:

A. Clotrimazole
B. Sytemic terbinafine
C. Itraconazole
D. Griseofulvin + Steroid

5. A patient has a non itchy plaque positive for hyphae, diagnosis is:
A. T capitis B. T corporis
C. T incognito D. T facei

6. All of the following drugs are effective in the treatment of pityriasis versicolor *except*:
A. Selenium sulphide B. Ketoconazole
C. Griseofulvin D. Clotrimazole

7. A 36 years old factory worker developed itchy, annular scaly plaques in both groins. Application of a corticosteroid ointment lead to temporary relief but the plaques continued to extend at the periphery. The most likely diagnosis is:
A. Erythema annulare centrifugum
B. Granuloma annulare
C. Annular lichen planus
D. Tinea cruris

8. A 22 years old male patient presents with complaints of severe itching and white scaly lesions in the groin for past month. Which of the following is most likely to be the causative agent?
A. Trichophyton rubrum
B. Candida albicans
C. Candida glabrata
D. Malassezia furfur

9. A 24 years old man had multiple, small hypopigmented macules on the upper chest and back for the last three months. The macules were circular, arranged around follicles and many had coalesced to form large sheets. The surface of the macules showed fine scaling. He had similar lesions one year ago which subsided with treatment. The most appropriate investigation to confirm the diagnosis is:
A. Potassium hydroxide preparation of scales
B. Slit skin smear from discrete macules
C. Tzanck test
D. Skin biopsy of coalesced macules

10. An 8 years old child has localized, non-cicatrical alopecia over scalp with itching and scales. The diagnosis is:
A. Tinea barbae B. Alopecia areata
C. Tinea capitis D. Lichen planus

11. An eleven years old boy is having tinea capitis on his scalp. The most appropriate line of treatment is:
A. Oral griseofulvin therapy
B. Topical griseofulvin therapy
C. Shaving of the scalp
D. Selenium sulphide shampoo

12. A 5-year-old boy has multiple asymtomatic oval and circular faintly hypopigmented macules with fine scaling on his face. The most probable clinical diagnosis is:
A. Ptyriasis versicolor
B. Indeterminate leprosy
C. Ptyriasis alba
D. Acrofacial vitiligo

13. Most common organisim causing tinea capitis is:
A. Trichophyton tonsurans
B. Microsporum
C. Epidermophyton
D. Candida albicans

14. Chandu a 30 years male presents with alopecia, boggy scalp swelling and easily pluckable hair. Diagnostic test is:
A. KOH smear B. Culture sensitivity
C. Biopsy D. None

15. Tinea capitis is caused by all *except*:
A. Epidermophyton B. Microsporum
C. T. violaceum D. T. schoenleinii

16. Black dot ring worm is caused by:
A. Microsporon B. Trichophyton
C. Epidiermophyton D. Candida

17. Tinea capitis is not caused by:
A. Microsporum canis
B. Trichophyton mentagrophyte
C. Epidermophyton
D. Trichophyton rubrum

18. Wood's lamp negative with a grey patch is caused by:
A. Microsporum canis
B. Trichophyton mentagrophyte
C. Epidermophyton
D. Trichophyton rubrum

19. Hair perforation test is done for:
A. Microsporum canis
B. Trichophyton mentagrophyte
C. Epidermophyton
D. Trichophyton rubrum

20. The following is an endothrix infection:
A. Microsporum canis
B. Trichophyton mentagrophyte
C. Epidermophyton
D. Trichophyton tonsurans

Answers :

1. C	2. C	3. D	4. D
5. C	6. C	7. B	8. A
9. A	10. C	11. A	12. C
13. B	14. B	15. A	16. B
17. C,D	18. B	19. B	20. D

BACTERIAL, LEPROSY, TUBERCULOSIS

1. A 7 years old child presenting with recurrent dry scaly macules (White small) on face has:
A. Indeterminate leprosy
B. Post dermal leishmaniasis
C. Pityriasis alba
D. Thalidomide

2. Erythema nodosum leprosum occurs in:
A. Lepromatous leprosy
B. Tuberculoid leprosy
C. Boderline lepromatous
D. Boderline tuberculoid

3. Treatment of lepra type II reaction are all *except*:
A. Clofazimine
B. Thalidomide
C. Corticosteroids
D. Antileprosy treatment
E. Cessation of antileprosy treatment

4. Erythrasma is caused by:
A. Corynebacterium minutissimum
B. Diphtheriae
C. C. ulceranans
D. C. vaginale

5. Which of the following is not characterized by a plaque showing central scarring?
A. Lupus vulgaris B. TBVC
C. Baghdad boil D. DLE

6. Swimming pool granuloma is caused by: †
A. M. bovius B. M. ulcerans
C. M. kansaii D. M. balanei

Imp: M *marinum is the other cause*

7. Acute neuritis in leprosy responds best to:
A. Predinsolone B. Thalidomide
C. Clofazimine D. Dapsone

8. Earliest sensation to be lost in Hansen's disease is:†
A. Pain
B. Touch
C. Warm temperature
D. Cold temperature

9. Tuberculoid leprosy is characterised by all *except*:
A. Non caseating granuloma in nerve
B. Sub-epidermal free zone
C. Bacilli in skin
D. Skin caseation

10. Duration of treatment in pauci, bacillary leprosy is:
A. 6 months
B. 9 months
C. 2 years
D. Till sumptoms subside

11. The daily dose of thalidomide for controlling E.N.L. is:
A. 100 mg B. 200–300 mg
C. 500 mg D. 1000 mg only

12. The most sensitive parameter to assess the drug effectiveness in the skin smears of leprosy †patients is:
A. Bacteriological index
B. Morphological index
C. Granuloma index
D. None of the above

13. Reversal lepra reaction shows no response to:
A. Clofazimine B. Chloroquine
C. Glucocorticoids D. Thalidomide

14. Most common nerve involved in leprosy:
A. Ulnar B. Median
C. Radial D. Musculocutaneous

15. Drug of choice with type I lepra reaction with severe neuritis is:

A. Prednisolone B. Clofazimine
C. Thalidomide D. Chloroquine

16. One of the following is a side effect of clofazimine used in leprosy therapy:
A. Hyperpigmentation
B. Erythema
C. Discoloration of body secretions
D. Macular rash

17. About the treatment of paucibacillary leprosy the most preferred regimen is:
A. Dapsone 100 mg OD for 6 months
B. Dapsone 100 mg OD and Rifampicin 300 mg OD for 6 months
C. Dapsone 100 mg OD and Rifampicin 300 mg monthly for 6 months
D. Dapsone 100 mg OD and Rifampicin 600 mg monthly for 6 months

18. Which of the following is an indication of active leprosy? †
A. New skin lesions B. MI
C. Erythema D. BI

19. All of the following are true of tuberculoid leprosy *except*:
A. It is anaesthetic
B. Positive lepromin test
C. Treatment for 2 years
D. Body immunity is high

20. Lesion not seen in lepromatous leprosy is:
A. Macule B. Papule
C. Nodule D. Vesicle

21. Slit smear negative leprosy is:
A. Neuritic type B. Tuberculoid type
C. Indeterminate type D. Lepra reaction

22. Nerve abscess in tuberculoid leprosy treatment of choice: †††
A. Incision and drainage B. Clofazimine
C. Steroids D. Thalidomide

23. All are true about lepromatous leprosy *except*:
A. Presence of globi
B. Subepidermal free zone
C. Decreased cell mediated immunity
D. Presence of granulomas subdermally

24. Satellite lesion is seen in which leprosy?
A. Tuberculoid B. BT
C. IL D. Histoid leprosy

25. In leprosy neural involvement occurs in what percentage of patients? †
A. 30% B. 60%
C. 90% D. 100%

26. Most common type of leprosy in India: †
A. BT B. TT
C. IL D. BL

27. Sec. syphilis, true about rash is:
A. Pruritic B. Vesicular
C. Asymptomatic D. Tender

28. Leprosy does not involve: †††
A. CNS B. Testes
C. Skin D. Cornea

29. Staphylococcus causes all *except*:
A. Scarlet fever B. TSS
C. Carbuncle D. Sycosis barbae

30. Mycobacterium causing skin ulcer:
A. M. ulcerans B. M. fortuitum
C. M. marinum D. Butcher warts

31. Which of the following represents a variant of LL Hansen?
A. Histoid Hansen B. Lazarine leprosy
C. LMDF D. Acne agminata

32. In which classification does lepromin help in diagnosis? †
A. Ridley Jopling B. Indian
C. Madrid D. Administrative

33. In which leprosy is the lepromin test negative, inverted saucer is seen and biopsy reveals onion peel perineum?
A. BT B. TT
C. BL D. BB

34. Satellite lesion are seen in:
A. Tuberculoid leprosy
B. Lepromatous leprosy
C. Borderline tuberculoid leprosy
D. Histoid leprosy

35. Skin biopsy in leprosy is characterized by:
A. Periappendageal bacilli
B. Periappendageal lymphocytosis
C. Perivascular lymphocytosis
D. All of the above

36. Single lesion in skin is seen in which type of leprosy?
A. TT B. BT
C. BL D. LL

37. An 8 years old boy from Bihar presents with a 6 months history of an ill defined, hypopigmented slightly atrophic macule on the face. The most likely diagnosis is:
A. Pityriasis alba
B. Indeterminate leprosy
C. Morphea
D. Calcium deficiency

38. Lepromin test is positive in:
A. Lepromatous leprosy
B. Indeterminate leprosy
C. Tuberculoid leprosy
D. Histoid leprosy

39. Most potent anti leprotic drug is:
A. Clofazimine B. Dapsone
C. Rifampicin D. Norfloxacin

40. Anti leprotic drug used in lepra reaction is:
A. Acedapsone B. Rifampicin
C. Dapsone D. Clofazimine

41. A 20 years old male from Jaipur with erythematous lesion on cheek with central crusting likely diagnosis is:
A. SLE
B. Lupus vulgaris
C. Chillblain
D. Cutaneous leishmaniasis

42. Cutaneous tuberculosis secondary to underlying tissue is called as:
A. Lupus vulgaris
B. Scrofuloderma
C. Spina ventosa
D. Tuberculous verrucosa cutis

43. A 27-year-old patient was diagnosed to have borderline leprosy and started on multibacillary multi-drug therapy. Six weeks later, he developed pain in the nerves and redness and swelling of the skin lesions. The management of his illness should include all of the following, *except*:
A. Stop anti-leprosy drugs
B. Systemic corticosteroids
C. Rest to the limbs affected
D. Analgesics

44. A 16 years old student reported for the evaluation of multiple hypopigmented macules on the trunk and limbs. All of the following tests are useful in making a diagnosis of leprosy, *except*:
A. Sensation testing B. Lepromin test
C. Slit smears D. Skin biopsy

45. A 12 years old boy had a gradually progressive plaque on a buttock for the last 3 years. The plaque was 15 cm in diameter, annular in shape, with crusting and induration at the periphery and scarring at the center. The most likely diagnosis:
A. Tinea corporis
B. Granuloma annulare
C. Lupus vulgaris
D. Borderline leprosy

46. Best method for treatment of ulnar nerve abscess in a case of leprosy is: †††
A. Incision and drainage
B. High dose of steroid
C. Thalidomide
D. High dose of clofazimine

Answers :

1. C	2. A,C	3. E	4. A
5. C	6. C	7. A	8. D
9. B	10. A	11. B	12. B
13. D	14. A	15. A	16. C
17. D	18. B	19. C	20. D
21. A,C	22. C	23. D	24. B
25. D	26. C	27. C	28. A
29. A	30. A	31. A	32. A
33. C	34. C	35. D	36. A
37. B	38. C	39. C	40. D
41. D	42. B	43. A	44. B
45. C	46. B		

INFECTION

1. Which pyoderma afflicts the lower limb and heals with a scar?
A. Folliculitis B. Impetigo
C. Cellulitis D. Echthyma

2. **Sycosis barbae is a form of:**
   A. Pyoderma
   B. Folliculitis
   C. Fungal infection
   D. Lupus

3. **A dermatoses that is seen in immunosuppression with a count of CD_4^+ count less than 300 cells/mL is all *except*:**
   A. Eosinophilic folliculitis
   B. Ofuji disease
   C. Acne keloidalis nuchae
   D. Pseudofolliculitis barbae

4. **Which of the following is cause by corynebacterium minutissimum?**
   A. Erysepiloid
   B. Anthrax
   C. Trichomycosis axillaris
   D. Pitted keratolysis

5. **A condition that affects the genitourinary system with Michaelis-Gutmann bodies is called as:**
   A. Leukoplakia
   B. Zoons balanitis
   C. Erythroplasia of queret
   D. Malacoplakia

6. **Characteristic lesion of scabies seen in infants is:**
   A. Burrow
   B. Fissure
   C. Vesicle
   D. Papule

7. **Which of the following resident florae are incorrectly matched?**
   A. S. aureus: nares
   B. E. coli: ear
   C. Aerobic coliforms: perineum
   D. P acnes: axilla

Answers :

1. D	**2. A,B**	**3. C,D**	**4. C,D**
5. D	**6. C**	**7. C**	

INFESTATION

1. **Most severe form of scabies:**
   A. Norwegian scabies
   B. Nodular scabies
   C. Animal scabies
   D. Genital scabies

2. **The drug of choice for scabies is:**
   A. Sulphur ointment
   B. Benzyl benzoate
   C. Gamma benzene hexachloride
   D. Permethrin 5%

3. **The burrows in scabies is in the:**
   A. Straum germination
   B. S basale
   C. Straum corneum
   D. S lucidum

4. **Scabies in children differs from that in adults in that it affects:**
   A. Webs pace
   B. Face and scalp
   C. Genitalia
   D. Axilla

5. **Macula caerulae is seen in:**
   A. Pediculosis humanis corporis
   B. Pediculosis capitis
   C. Pthiris pubis
   D. Lupus erythematosis

6. **Incubation period of scabies is:**
   A. 7 days
   B. 2 weeks
   C. 4 weeks
   D. 2–3 days

7. **Vagabond's disease is:**
   A. Pediculosis corposis
   B. Scabies
   C. Eczema
   D. Ringworm

8. **An 8 months old child presented with itchy, exudative lesions on the face, palms and soles. The siblings also have similar complaints. The treatment of choice is such a patient is:**
   A. Systemic ampicillin
   B. Topical betamethasone
   C. Systemic prednisolone
   D. Topical permethrin

9. **An infant presenting with itchy lesions over groin and prepuce all is indicated *except*:**
   A. Bathe and apply scabicidal solution
   B. Treatment of all family members
   C. Dispose all clothes by burning
   D. I.V. antibiotics

10. **Rakesh, a 27-year-old boy had itchy, excoriated papules on the forehead and the exposed parts of the arms and legs for 3 years. The disease was most severe in the rainy season and improved completely in winter. The most likely diagnosis is:**

A. Insect bite hypersensitivity
B. Scabies
C. Urticaria
D. Atopic dermatitis

11. A child comes with itching on the scalp with occipital and post auricular enlarged lymph node the most likely diagnosis is:

A. Tinea capitis B. Scabies
C. Folliculitis D. P capitis

12. Plica polonica is seen in:

A. Tinea capitis B. Scabies
C. Folliculitis D. P capitis

13. Vagabond disease is another name for:

A. Tinea corporis B. Scabies
C. Dermatitis D. P corporis

14. Maculae cerulae is a classic sign seen in:

A. Tinea corporis B. Scabies
C. Dermatitis D. P corporis

15. Average number of mites seen in a patient are:

A. 3 B. 4
C. 50 D. 11

16. Treatment of cleanman scabies is:

A. Permethrin B. Steroids
C. Crotamiton D. D. lindane

Answers :

1. A	2. D	3. C	4. B
5. A	6. C	7. A	8. D
9. D	10. A	11. D	12. D
13. D	14. D	15. D	16. B

S.T.D.

1. Drug of choice for chancroid with HIV:

A. Azithromycin B. Ceftriaxone
C. Penicillin D. Erythromycin

2. Drug of choice for granuloma venereum:

A. Doxycyline B. Streptomycin
C. Penicillin D. Erythromycin

3. Drug of choice for gonorrhoea with chlamydia:

A. Azithromycin 2g B. Ceftriaxone
C. Streptomycin D. Sulphonamide

4. Hutchinson's syphilitic triad includes all *except*:

A. Associated with congenital syphilis
B. Notched incisor teeth
C. Nerve deafness
D. Interstitial keratitis
E. Associated with CVS anomalies

5. Most sensitive test in secondary stage treatment of syphillis:†

A. TPHA B. VDRL
C. FTAbs D. Capita-IgM ELISA

6. Pseudobuboes are found in:

A. Chancroid B. LGV
C. Granuloma inguinale D. All of the above

7. School of fish appearance is shown by:

A. Hemophilus ducreyi
B. Gonococcus
C. Chlamydia
D. Donovania granulomatis

8. Safety pin appearance is shown by:

A. Hemophilus ducreyi
B. Chlamydia
C. Donovani granulomatis
D. Mycoplasma

9. Sign of groove is found in:

A. Chancroid
B. Granuloma inguinale
C. LGV
D. Syphilis

10. Most infectious manifestation of secondary syphilis is:

A. Lymphadenopathy
B. Rash
C. Snail track ulcer
D. Condylomata lata

11. Esthiomine is seen in:

A. Chancroid B. Syphilis
C. LGV D. Gonorrhoea

12. Podophyllin is used in:

A. Condyloma lata
B. Condyloma acuminata
C. Palmar warts
D. Plantar warts

13. Treponema pallidum crosses placenta:

A. After 36 weeks
B. After 28 weeks
C. After 16 weeks
D. At any stage of pregnancy

14. A 20 years old male developed multiple tender non-indurated bleeding ulcers over prepuce 4 days after sexual exposure. The most probable diagnosis in this patient is:

A. Primary syphilis
B. Lymphogranuloma venereum
C. Chancroid
D. Donovanosis

15. Genital ulcer is not seen in:

A. LGV B. GI
C. Syphilis D. Chancroid

16. Condyloma lata is present in syphilis in:

A. Primary B. Secondary
C. Tertiary D. Latent

17. To indicate effective therapy in syphilis VDRL test should have a fall in titre of: †

A. One fold B. Two folds
C. Three folds D. Four folds

18. Treatment of both partners is recommended in all *except*:

A. Candida infection
B. Gardenella
C. Herpes
D. Trichomonas vaginalis

19. Which of the following test is preferred for diagnosing congenital syphilis? †

A. VDRL B. TPHA
C. IgM FTAbs D. TPI

20. Drug of choice for P pubis:

A. Ivermectin B. BHC
C. Permethrin D. Crotomiton

21. True about syphilis is all *except*:

A. VDRL is sensitive but not specific
B. Infection leads to life long immunity
C. IgM and IgA antibodies are involved
D. T. pallidium when inoculated in rabbit produce progressive disease

22. Buboes with multiple sinuses discharging into inguinal lymph nodes are seen in:

A. Chancroid
B. Granuloma inguinale
C. LGV
D. Syphilis

23. The syndrome management of urethral discharge includes treatment of:

A. Neisseria gonorrhoeae and herpes genitalis
B. Chlamydia trachomatis and herpes genitalis
C. Neisseria gonorrhea and chlamydia trachomatis
D. Syphilis and chancroid

24. The most frequent cause of recurrent genital ulceration in a sexually active male is:

A. Herpes genitalis B. Aphthous ulcer
C. Syphilis D. Chancroid

25. Incorrect statement is:

A. VDRL titre decrease with treatment
B. VDRL becomes positive after 21 days of infection
C. FTA-ABS is earliest and most sensitive test
D. Yaws and Pinta can be defferentiated by serological tests

26. Genital elephantiasis is caused by:

A. Donovanosis
B. Congenital syphilis
C. Herpes genitalis
D. Lymphogranuloma venerum

27. A 19 years male develops painless penile ulcers 9 days after sexual intercourse with a professional sex worker likely diagnosis is:

A. Chancroid
B. Herpes
C. Chancre
D. Traumatic ulcer

28. A 30 years old male patient has a large, spreading and exuberant ulcer with bright red granulation tissue over the glans penis. There was no lymphadenopathy. The most likely causative organism is:

A. Treponema pallidum
B. Herpes simplex virus type 1
C. Herpes simplex virus type 2
D. Calymmatobacterium granulomatis

29. **A 24 years old male presents to an STD clinic with a single painless ulcer on external genitalia. The choice of laboratory test to look for the etiological agent would be:**
    A. Scrappings from ulcer for culture on chocolate agar with antibiotic supplement
    B. Serology for detection of specific IgM antibodies
    C. Scrappings from ulcer for dark field microscopy
    D. Scrappings from ulcer for tissue culture

30. **A 20 years old male develops multiple ulcer over prepuce and glans, which are painful along with suppurative inguinal lymphadenopathy, 5 days after having sexual intercourse with a lady, most probable diagnosis is:**
    A. Molluscum contagiosum
    B. Anaerobic streptococci
    C. Herpes
    D. Chancroid

31. **Culture positivity in chancroid is seen in:**
    A. 20% B. 30%
    C. 40% D. 60%

32. **According to NACO guidelines treatment of syphilis and chancroid with erythromycin is for:**
    A. 7 days B. 10 days
    C. 30 days D. 14 days

33. **The most common type of herpes genitalis is:**
    A. Asymptomatic
    B. First episode
    C. Recurrent
    D. Concomitant with other STD

34. **In primary herpes genitalis the viral shedding lasts for .... weeks.**
    A. 1 B. 2
    C. 3 D. 4

35. **LGV is diagnosed by complement fixation titre of >:**
    A. 1:8 B. 1:16
    C. 1:32 D. 1:512

36. **In syphilis FTA-IgM is positive after .... weeks. †**
    A. 1 B. 2
    C. 3 D. 4

37. **The positivity in secondary syphilis of VDRL is .... %.**
    A. 30 B. 40
    C. 50 D. 100

38. **Active infection in syphilis is diagnosed by a titre of VDRL >: †**
    A. 1:8 B. 1:16
    C. 1:32 D. I :512

39. **A patient of syphilis is given procain penicillin and develops hallucination and fits few minutes after the injection. This is called:**
    A. Jarisch herxheimer Rn
    B. Hypersensitivity reaction
    C. Hoignes reaction
    D. Serum sickness

40. **Bowenoid papulosis is caused by HPV types:**
    A. 1, 2 B. 3, 4
    C. 16, 18 D. 16

Answers :

1. D	2. A	3. A	4. E
5. D	6. C	7. A	8. C
9. C	10. D	11. C	12. B
13. C	14. C	15. A	16. B
17. D	18. B, A	19. C	20. C
21. C, D	22. C	23. C	24. A
25. C, D	26. D	27. C	28. D
29. C	30. D	31. B	32. D
33. A	34. A	35. D	36. A
37. D	38. B	39. C	40. D

HIV

1. **Which of the following drugs are effective in the treatment of herpes simplex resistant to acyclovir?**
    A. Acyclovir B. Corticosteroids
    C. Interferons D. Foscarnet

2. **The most frequent causative organisms for nongonococcal urethritis include:**
    A. Chlamydia trachomatis
    B. Staphylococcus saprophyticus
    C. Ureaplasma urealyticum
    D. All of the above

3. **Which of the following is not true for atypical mycobacterium in HIV infection?**

A. Most commonly M avium-intracellulare-complex
B. Usually CD4 less than 200
C. Macrolide, ethambutol
D. ATT can be given

4. **Which about the treatment of bacillary angiomatosis is not true?**
A. < CD 4–100
B. Erythromycin
C. Clofazimine
D. Steroids

5. **Which of the following are specific dermatoses of HIV *except*:**
A. Exanthem of acute retroviral syndrome
B. PSO (proximal subungual onychomycoses)
C. OHL (oral hairy leucoplakia)
D. Seborrheic dermatitis, xerosis

6. **Which of the following drugs are useful in treating histoplasmosis?**
A. Amph B 0.7 mg/kg I.V. OD 2 week
B. Griseofulvin
C. Fluconazole
D. Flucytosine

7. **Which of the following drugs are useful in treating psoriasis in HIV *except?***
A. HAART B. PUVA
C. Retinoids D. Steroids

Answers :			
1. C,D	2. A	3. D	4. D
5. D	6. A	7. D	

Section 3

DERMATITIS

1. **Most common site of atopic dermatitis in an inafant is:**
A. Scalp B. Elbow
C. Trunk D. Ant. cubital fossa

2. **Erythema pernio is due to:**
A. Heat B. Cold
C. Contact dermatitis D. Atopic dermatitis

3. **Most common metal causing skin hypersenitivity:**
A. Nickel B. Cu
C. Iron D. Brass

4. **Most common site of atopic dermatitis in a child aged 9 years is:**
A. Scalp B. Elbow
C. Trunk D. Ant. cubital fossa

5. **Berloque dermatitis is due to contact with:**
A. Metals B. Cosmetics
C. Food D. Plants

6. **Most common cause of air borne contact dematitis is:**
A. Crysanthemum B. Parthenium
C. Calotropis D. Bourgainvilla

7. **A 25 years old man presents with recurrent episodes of flexural eczema, contact urticaria, recurrent skin infections and severe abdominal cramps and diarrhoea upon taking sea foods. He is suffering from:**
A. Seborrheic dermatitis
B. Atopic dermatitis
C. Airborne contact dermatitis
D. Nummular dermatitis

8. **Most common cause of contact dermatitis in Indian females is:**
A. Vegetables
B. Nail polish remover
C. Nail polish
D. Detergents

9. **The sources of common allergens in hair dye is:**
A. Nickel
B. Co
C. Gold
D. Paraphenyleaminediamine

10. **Which of the following shows a white dermographism?**
A. Atopic dermatitis
B. Seborrheic dermatitis
C. Pomphylox
D. Psoriasis

11. **Which of the following is the most common cause of *contact dermatitis*? ††**
A. Water B. Ni
C. Co D. AU

It is important to understand – it means most common cause of ICD.

12. Sago grain appearance is seen in:

A. Atopic dermatitis
B. Seborrheic dermatitis
C. Pomphylox
D. Psoriasis

13. Most common cause of housewife dermatitis is:

A. Detergents B. Soap
C. Jewellery D. Vegetables

Answers :

1. A	2. B	3. A	4. D
5. B	6. B	7. B	8. D
9. D	10. A	11. A	12. C
13. A			

Section 4

CT DISORDERS/BULLOUS DISORDER

1. A girl of 19 years with arthritis and photosensitive rash on cheeks, likely diagnosis is:

A. SLE
B. Chlosma
C. Stevens-Johnson syndrome
D. Lyme's disease

2. Palpable pupura is seen in all conditions *except*:

A. Cryoglobulinemia
B. H.S. purpura
C. Giant cell arteritis
D. Drug induced vasculitis

3. A 40 years old woman presented with 8 months history of erythema and swelling of the periobital region and papules and plaques on the dorsolateral aspect of forearms and knuckles with ragged cuticles. There was no muscle weakness. The most likely diagnosis is:

A. Systemic lupus erythematosus
B. Dermatomyositis
C. Systemic sclerosis
D. Mixed connective tissue disorder

4. Toxic epidermal necrolysis is also called:

A. Sweet's syndrome
B. Lyell's syndrome
C. Hailey and Hailey's disease
D. Duhring's disease

5. Most common site of herpes gestationis is:

A. Periumbilical region B. Flanks of abdomen
C. Vulva D. Infraorbital

6. The treatment of dermatitis herpetiformis is:

A. Gluten free diet with minerals and vitamins
B. Carbamazepine
C. Acyclovir
D. Corticosteroids

7. Drug of choice for dermatitis herpetiformis is:

A. Dapsone B. Methotrexate
C. Clotrimazole D. Thiobendazole

8. Subepidermal bulla are seen in:

A. Bullous pemphigoid B. Pemphigus
C. Pityriasis rosea D. Psoriasis

9. Rarest variety of pemphigus is:

A. P. vulgaris B. P. foliaceus
C. P. vegetans D. P. erythematosis

10. Subepidermal blistering is seen in all *except*:

A. Pemphigus vulgairs
B. Dermatitis herpetiformis
C. Toxic epidermal necrolysis
D. Bullous pemphigoid
E. Hailey-Hailey disease

11. A 40 years old male reported with recurrent episodes of oral ulcers, large areas of denuded skin and flaccid vesiculobullous eruptions. Which is the most important bed-side investigation in establishing the diagnosis?

A. Gram-staining of the blister fluid
B. Culture and sensitivity
C. Skin biopsy and immunofluorescence
D. Tzanck smear from the floor of bulla

12. Acantholysis is seen in:

A. Epidermis
B. Dermis
C. Dermo-epidermjunction
D. Subcutaneous tissue

13. A 50 years old man has a 2 years history of facial bullae and oral ulcers. Microscopic smear from skin lesions is most likely to disclose:

A. Tzanck cells B. Acantholytic cells
C. Necrosis D. Koilocytosis

14. All are vesiculobullous lesions *except*:

A. Dermatitis herpetiformis B. Scabies
C. Pemphigus D. Pemphigoid

15. Acantholytic cells in pemphigus is:

A. Cell with hyperchromatic nuclei and perinuclear halo
B. Cell with hypochromatic nuclei and perinuclear halo
C. Multinucleated cells
D. None of the above

16. Etiology of epidermolysis bullosa is:

A. Genetic B. Infections
C. Senile D. Malignant
E. Metabolic

17. In pemphigus vulgaris, antibodies are present against:

A. Basement membrane
B. Intercellular substance
C. Cell nucleus
D. Keratin

18. A 30 years old male had severely itchy papula vesicular lesions on extremities, knees, elbows and buttocks for one year. Direct immunofluorescence staining of the lesions showed IgA deposition at dermoepiderma junction. The most probable diagnosis is:

A. Pemphigus vulgaris
B. Bullous pemphigoid
C. Dermatitis herpetiformis
D. Numinulareczema

19. A 40 years old male developed persistent oral ulcers followed by multiple flaccid bullae on trunk and extremities. Direct examination of a skin biopsy immunofluorescence showed intercellular IgG deposits in the epidermis:

A. Pemphigus vulgaris
B. Bullous pemphigoid
C. Bullous lupus erthematosus
D. Epidermolysis bullosa acquisita

20. A patient with bullous eruption on lower limb and trunk, biopsy show subepidermal bullae. The correct diagnosis is:

A. Pemphigoid B. Pemphigus vulgaris
C. Impetigo D. Internal malignancy

21. A 40 years old male had multiple blisters over the trunk and extremities. Direct immunofluorescence studies showed linear IgG deposits along the basement membrane. Which of the following is the most likely diagnosis?

A. Pemphigus vulgaris
B. Pemphigus foliaceous
C. Bullous pemphigoid
D. Dermatitis herpetiformis

22. A 24 years old female has flaccid bullae in the skin and oral erosions. Histopathology shows intraepidermal acantholytic blister. The most likely diagnosis is:

A. Pemphigoid
B. Erythema multiforme
C. Pemphigus vulgaris
D. Dermatitis herpetiformis

23. A 28 years old patient has multiple grouped papilovesicular lesions on bow elbows, knees, buttocks and upper back associated with severe itching. The most likely diagnosis is:

A. Pemphigus vulgaris
B. Bullous pemphigoid
C. Dermatitis herpetiformis
D. Herpes zoster

24. In an 8 days old child with no history of consanguinity in the parents, the mother reports blisters and bleeding off of the skin at the site of handling and pressure. There was a similar history in the previous child which proved to be fatal. The diagnosis is:

A. Bullous pemphigoid
B. Congenital syphilis
C. Congenital epidermolysis bullosa
D. Letterer-Siwe disease

25. Intra epidermal bulla is seen in:

A. Pemphigoid
B. Pemphigus
C. Dermatitis herpetiformis
D. Light reaction

Answers :

1. A	2. C	3. B	4. B	5. A,B
6. A	7. A	8. A	9. D	10. A,E
11. D	12. A	13. B	14. B	15. A
16. A	17. B	18. C	19. A	20. A
21. C	22. C	23. C	24. C	25. B

VASCULAR DERMATOSES

1. **Which of the following is a granulomatous vasculitis?**
   A. Essential mixed cryoglobulinemia
   B. Hyperglobulinemic purpuras (Waldenström's macroglobulinemia)
   C. Rheumatic vasculitis
   D. Churg-Strauss syndrome

2. **Which of the following is not a feature of Churg-Strauss syndrome?**
   A. Asthma
   B. Eosinophilia (>10%)
   C. E nodosum
   D. Chest X-ray showing nodules, infiltrates

3. **Which of the following is not a feature of takayasu arteritis:**
   A. BP >10 mmHg difference between two arms
   B. Bruits
   C. Neuropathy
   D. Hypertension (Diastolic BP >90 mm Hg)

4. **New headache with raised ESR is seen in:**
   A. Giant cell (temporal) arteritis (CGA)
   B. Takayasu's arteritis (TA)
   C. Polyarteritis nodosa (PAN)
   D. Wegener's granulomatosis (WG)

5. **Limb claudication and decreased brachial artery pulses are seen in:**
   A. Giant cell (temporal) arteritis (CGA)
   B. Takayasu's arteritis (TA)
   C. Polyarteritis nodosa (PAN)
   D. Wegener's granulomatosis (WG)

6. **Neuropathy, hypertension (diastolic BP >90 mm Hg) and renal impairment is seen in:**
   A. Giant cell (temporal) arteritis (CGA)
   B. Takayasu's arteritis (TA)
   C. Polyarteritis nodosa (PAN)
   D. Wegener's granulomatosis (WG)

7. **Asthma and eosinophilia (>10%) is seen in:**
   A. Churg-Strauss syndrome (CSS)
   B. Giant cell (temporal) arteritis (CGA)
   C. Takayasu's arteritis (TA)
   D. Polyarteritis nodosa

8. **Abdominal pain followed by purpura on the lower limb with IgA deposit in the kidney is seen in:**
   A. Henoch-Schönlein purpura (HSP)
   B. Giant cell (temporal) arteritis (CGA)
   C. Takayasu's arteritis (TA)
   D. Polyarteritis nodosa

Answers :

1. A	2. C	3. C,D	4. A
5. B	6. C	7. A	8. A

Section 5

PAPULOSQUAMOUS DERMATOSES

1. **Koebner's phenomenon is seen in:**
   A. Lichen planus
   B. Psoriasis
   C. Icthyosis
   D. Pityriasis rubra pilaris

2. **All are common of psoriasis *except*:**
   A. Nail changes
   B. Extensor distribution
   C. Arthritis
   D. Oral mucosa

3. **The treatment of psoriatic erythroderma is:**
   A. Methotrexate B. Retinoids
   C. Dithranol D. Corticosteroid

4. **'Fir-tree' type of distribution is seen in:**
   A. Pityriasis rosea B. Psoriasis
   C. Measles D. Secondary syphilis

5. **A 30 years old male present with pruritic flat-topped polygonal, shiny violaceous papules with flexural distribution. The most likely diagnosis is:**
   A. Psoriasis
   B. Pityriasis rosea
   C. Lichen planus
   D. Lichenoid dermatitis

6. **Psoriasis is exacerbated by:**
   A. Lithium B. β-blockers
   C. Anti-malarials D. All of the above

7. **The important fearure of psoriasis is:**
   A. Crusting B. Scaling
   C. Oozing D. Erythema

8. **Most characteristic feature of lichen planus is all *except*:**
   A. Thinning of nail plate is most common
   B. Non scarring alopecia
   C. Violaceous lesions on skin and mucous membrane
   D. Wickham striae

9. **The most characteristic finding in lichen planus is: ††**
   A. Civatte bodies
   B. Basal cell degeneration
   C. Thinning of nail plate
   D. Violaceous lesions

10. **Which of the following statements is true regarding pityriasis rubra pilaris:**
    A. Isolated patches of normal skin are found
    B. Cephalocaudal distribution
    C. More common in females
    D. Oral cyclosporine is effective

11. **A 16 years old presented with asymptomatic, multiple, erythematous annular lesions with a collarette of scales at the periphery of the lesions present on the trunk. The most likely diagnosis is:**
    A. Pityriasis versicolor   B. Pityriasis alba
    C. Pityriasis rosea   D. Pityriasis pilaris

12. **The only definite indication for giving systemic corticosteroids in pustular psoriasis is:**
    A. Psoriatic erythroderma with pregnancy
    B. Psoriasis in a patient with alcoholic cirrhosis
    C. Moderate arthritis
    D. Extensive lesions

13. **Exfoliative dermatitis can be due to all of the following diseases *except*:**
    A. Drug hypersensitivity
    B. Pityriasis rubra pilaris
    C. Pityriasis rosea
    D. Psoriasis

14. **A patient with psoriasis was started on systemic steroids. After stopping treatment, the patient developed generalized pustules all over the body. The cause is most likely to be:**
    A. Drug induced reaction
    B. Pustular psoriasis
    C. Bacterial infections
    D. Septicemia

15. **All are true regarding psoriasis *except*:**
    A. Arthritis in 5%
    B. Micro Munro abscess are seen
    C. Head, neck and face are not involved
    D. Non scaly, red lesions are seen in inframammary and natal area

16. **Regarding lichen planus all are true *except*:**
    A. Hypopigmentation in residual disease
    B. Lymphocytic infiltration in supradermal layer
    C. Itchy, polygonal, purple, papule
    D. Skin, hair and oral mucosa commonly involved

17. **A patient presents with scarring alopecia, thinned nails, hypopigmented macular lesions over trunk and oral mucosa. The diagnosis is:**
    A. Psoriasis   B. Leprosy
    C. Lichen planus   D. Pemphigus

18. **A checkerboard pattern on histology is seen in:**
    A. Psoriasis   B. Lichen planus
    C. PRP   D. Atopic dermatitis

19. **Which of the following can go into mycoses fungoides?**
    A. PLC
    B. PLEVA
    C. Large plaque parapsoriasis
    D. Psoriasis

Answers :

1. A, B	2. D	3. A	4. A
5. C	6. D	7. B, D	8. B
9. C	10. A, B	11. C	12. A
13. C	14. B	15. C	16. A
17. C	18. C	19. C	

Section 6

DISORDER OF PIGMENTATION

1. **An increased incidence of vitiligo is found in:**
   A. Diabetes mellitus
   B. Nutritional deficiency
   C. Old age
   D. Psoriasis

2. **Slate like discoloration of the skin is caused by all these drugs *except*:**
   A. Chlorpromazine   B. Minocycline
   C. Amiodarone   D. Thiacetazone

3. In a patch of vitiligo:
A. Melanin synthesis is inhibited
B. Melanosomes are absent
C. Melanocytes are absent
D. Melanocytes are reduced

4. Riehl's melanosis mainly invloves:
A. Face and neck B. Trunk
C. Extremities D. Palms only

5. Rain drop pigmentation is seen in:
A. Chronic lead poisoning
B. Chronic arsenic poisoning
C. Chronic mercury poisoning
D. All of the above

6. A child presents with a solitary white well defined patch on his right thigh. What is the diagnosis?
A. Piebaldism B. Acral vitiligo
C. Nevus achromicus D. Albinism

7. Babloo, a 4 years old boy, presents with history of seizures, on examination there is hypopigmented patches on his face. There is mental retardation also. What is most likely diagnosis?
A. Neurofibromatosis
B. Tuberous sclerosis
C. Sturge-Weber syndrome
D. Incontinentia pigmenti

Answers :

1. A	2. B	3. C	4. A
5. B	6. C	7. B	

PIGMENTARY

1. What is the melanocyte keratinocyte ratio?
A. 1:1 B. 1:10
C. 1:28 D. 1:36

2. What is the topical macrolide used in vitiligo?
A. Tacrolimus B. Calcipotriol
C. Tazarotene D. Meanocyl

3. Diascopy is used for:
A. N anemicus B. N depigmentosus
C. Vitiligo D. Melasma

4. Which of the following is not used for melasma?
A. Steroids B. Hydroquinone
C. Tretinoin D. Laser

5. All are seen in tuberous sclerosis *except*:
A. Iris nodule
B. Renal cortical cyst
C. Rhabdomyoma of heart and lung
D. Adenoma sebaceum

6. Inheritence of icthyosis vulgaris is:
A. X-linked dominant
B. X-linked recessive
C. Autosomal dominant
D. Autosomal recessive

Answers :

1. D	2. A	3. A	4. D
5. A	6. C		

Section 7

SKIN CANCER

1. Which of the following does not have lymphatic spread?
A. Squamous cell carcinoma
B. Basal cell carcinoma
C. Malignant melanoma
D. Adenocarcinoma

2. Which naevi commonly predisposes to malignant melanoma?
A. Dermal B. Junctional
C. Congenital D. Lentigo

3. Treatment of choice in solar keratosis/active keratosis:
A. Methotrexate
B. Topical 5 FU
C. Topical mechlorethamine
D. Chemosurgery

4. Following is true about freckles *except*:
A. Age of onset is 7-8 years
B. Bilateral symmetrical on exposed parts and increase on exposure
C. Prone to malignancy
D. Familial

5. Changes of squamous cell carcinoma are seen in:
A. Seborrheic keratosis B. Bowen's disease
C. Lichen planus D. OIE

6. Lisch nodule is seen in:
A. Von Recklinghausen's disease
B. Lupus vulgaris
C. Leprosy
D. LGV

7. Genodermal disease that can cause skin malignancy are:
A. Xeroderma pigmentosa
B. Neurofibromatosis
C. Actinic keratosis
D. Porphyria cutanea tarda

Answers :

1. B	2. C	3. B	4. C
5. B	6. A	7. A	

Section 8

ALOPECIA

1. Non-cicatrical alopecia is present in:
A. Scleroderma
B. Lichen planus
C. Psoriasis
D. Kerion

2. Alopecia areata is treated by:
A. Minoxidil
B. Tranquilizers
C. Whitfields oinment
D. Parenteral penicillin

3. Alopecia areata is due to:
A. Estrogen stimulation
B. Androgen stimulation
C. Lichenoid reaction
D. Auto immune

4. Pseudo pelade is synonym of:
A. Alopecia steatoides
B. Premature alopecia
C. Traction
D. Cicatricial alopecia

5. The time period that elapses between the physical or emotional stress and the hair loss is about:
A. 21 days
B. 30 days
C. 3 months
D. 6 months

6. In alopecia areata, seen in:
A. Exclamatory mark hair
B. Scaring
C. Fungal infection
D. Traumatic

7. Cicatricial alopecia is seen in:
A. Lichen planus
B. DLE
C. Psoriasis
D. Alopecia areata
E. SLE

8. Contraindicated in androgenic alopecia:
A. Testosterone
B. Minoxidil
C. Cyproterone
D. Finasteride

9. Which of the following is a new drug to treat hirsutism?
A. Chemical depilatories
B. Bleaching agents
C. Nd-Yag laser
D. Eflornithine hydrochloride

10. The normal anagen to telogen ratio is:
A. 12:1
B. 5:1
C. 1:12
D. 1:5

11. Which of the following is a cause of scarring alopecia?
A. Discoid lupus
B. Alopecia areata
C. Lichen planus
D. Anagen effluvium

12. Which of the following is associated with increased hair fragility?
A. Monilethrix
B. Trichorrhexis nodosa
C. Anagen effluvium
D. Alopecia areata

13. Which of the following are seen in adult females only?
A. Lanugo hairs
B. Vellus
C. Terminal hairs
D. Kenogen hair

14. A patient is on chemotherapy and complains of hair loss, this is called:
A. Anagen effluvium
B. Alopecia areata
C. Telogen effluvium
D. Trichorrhexis nodosa

Answers :

1. C	2. A	3. D	4. D
5. C	6. A	7. A/B	8. A
9. D	10. A	11. C,A	12. A,B
13. B	14. A		

ACNE VULGARIS

1. Rhinophyma is:

A. Glandular form of acne rosacea
B. Form of acne vulgaris
C. Affects the scalp
D. A form of dermatofibroma

2. Acne vulgaris is caused by:

A. Staph aureus
B. Diphtheroids
C. Sweat gland hyperplasia
D. Obstruction to pilosebaceous duct

3. Crystaline miliaria is due to obstruction to:

A. Sebaceous glands
B. Sweat glands
C. Hair roots
D. Accessory sweat glands

4. The concentration of hydroquinone for treating cholasma should be:

A. 1%
B. 1 to 2%
C. 2 to 5%
D. 100

5. Treatment of acne vulgaris may include all *except*:

A. Cryotherapy
B. Oestrogens
C. UV light
D. Androgens

6. Comedones are characteristics of:

A. Acne vulgaris
B. Acne rosasea
C. SLE
D. Adenoma sebaeceum

7. Acne vulgaris invloves:

A. Pilosebaceous gland
B. Sebaceous gland
C. Eccrine gland
D. Apocrine gland

8. A 40 years old woman presents with a 2 years history of erythematous papulopustular lesions on the convexities of the face. There is a background of erythema and telangiectasia. The most likely diagnosis in the patient is:

A. Acne vulgaris
B. Rosacea
C. Systemic lupus erythematosus
D. Polymorphic light eruption

Answers :

1. A	2. D	3. B	4. C
5. D	6. A	7. A	8. B

Section 9

PEDIATRIC DERMATOLOGY

1. A child comes at 2 weeks with pustules on the groin, which do not have neutrophils or eosinophils, the most likely cause is:

A. Acropustulosis of infancy
B. Eosinophilic pustular folliculitis
C. Erythema toxicum
D. Candidiasis

2. A full term baby comes with generalized pustules which have eosinophils in them. The diagnosis is:

A. Acropustulosis of infancy
B. Eosinophilic pustular folliculitis
C. Erythema toxicum
D. Miliaria putulsosis

3. A 6 months old child comes with pustules on the scalp which have eosinophils in them. The diagnosis is:

A. Transient neonatal pustular melanosis
B. Acropustulosis of infancy
C. Eosinophilic pustular folliculitis
D. Erythema toxicum

4. A 1 month old child has high grade fever and comes with red itchy papules all over the body, the diagnosis is:

A. Transient neonatal pustular melanosis
B. Acropustulosis of infancy
C. Eosinophilic pustular folliculitis
D. Miliaria rubra

5. "Systemic disease fish-mouth" scars are seen in:

A. Ehlers-Danlos syndrome
B. Pseudoxanthoma elasticum
C. Scleroderma
D. Sarcoidosis

Answers :

1. D	2. C	3. C	4. D	5. A

SYSTEMIC DISEASE

1. Which of the following is a sign associated with microangiopathy in diabetes?

A. Necrobiosis lipoidica diabeticorum
B. Diabetic dermopathy
C. Granuloma annulare
D. Tinea

2. **"A wood-grain" pattern is seen in:**
   A. Erythema annulare
   B. Erythema multiforme
   C. Erythema chronicum migrans
   D. Erythema gyratum repens

3. **Necrolytic migratory erythema is a sign of underlying cancer due to involvement of:**
   A. Liver
   B. Kidney
   C. Testis
   D. Pancreas

4. **Hyper pigmentation mainly in flexure, and of nail is seen in:**
   A. Vitamin A deficiency
   B. Vitamin B_6 deficiency
   C. Vitamin B_{12} deficiency
   D. Vitamin B_3 deficiency

5. **In which condition do you see the glove and gauntlet sign?**
   A. Pellagra B. Phrynoderma
   C. Marasmus D. Kwashiorkor

6. **Barlow's disease is because of deficiency of:**
   A. Vitamin A B. Vitamin B
   C. Vitamin D D. Vitamin C

Answers :

1. A, B	2. D	3. D	4. C
5. A	6. D		

MISCELLANEOUS

1. **Darier's sign is seen in:**
   A. Xenoderma pigmentosa
   B. Urticaria pigmentosa
   C. Herpes zoster
   D. Glucogonoma

2. **Chloroquine is used in the treatment of:**
   A. DLE
   B. Pemphigus
   C. Psoriasis
   D. Nummular eczema

3. **Mast cell is stained by:**
   A. Giemsa B. Silver nitrate
   C. PAS D. Toluidine blue

4. **"Cayenne Pepper" stippling due to hemosiderin is found in:**
   A. Erythroplasia of queyrat
   B. Paget's disease
   C. Zoon's balanitis
   D. Pigmented purpuric destimatosis

5. **Acantholysis is seen in:**
   A. Pemphigus
   B. Pemphigoid
   C. Psoriasis
   D. Stevens-Johnson syndrome

6. **Drug of choice in herpes zoster:**
   A. Acyclovir B. Vidarabine
   C. Idoxuridine D. Actinomycin

7. **Photochemotherapy is used in the treatment of:**
   A. Pityriasis rosea B. Erythroderma
   C. Psoriasis D. Scabies

8. **Ballooning is characteristic of:**
   A. Herpes zoster B. Pemphigus
   C. Pemphigoid D. Insect bite

9. **Nail involvement is not a feature of:**
   A. Dermatophytosis B. Lichen planus
   C. DLE D. Psoriasis

10. **Degeneration of basal cells occurs in:**
    A. Lichen planus B. Pemphigus
    C. Psoriasis D. Pamphigoid

11. **Gottron's papules or sign is seen in:**
    A. Dermatomyositis B. Multiple myeloma
    C. Acute myeloid leukemia D. Psoriasis

12. **'Slapped cheeks' appearance is seen in:**
    A. Roseloa infantum
    B. Erythema subitum
    C. Erythema infectiosum
    D. Erythema multiforme

13. **A reticular pattern of cutaneous vasodilation is seen in:**
    A. Cutis marmorata B. Livedo reticularis
    C. Fifth disease D. All of the above

14. **'Honey colored' crusts are characteristic of:**
    A. Nummulareczema B. Impetigo
    C. Herpes zoster D. Cutaneous diphtheria

15. Bromhidrosis may be produced by intake of the following *except*:

A. Sounf B. Ginger
C. Onions D. Garlic

16. Fordyce's disease mainly involves:

A. Lips B. Buccal mucosa
C. Neck D. Trunk

17. Acrodermatitis enteropathica responds dramatically to:

A. Corticosteroids B. Dapsone
C. Zinc D. Ciprofloxacin

18. Oil drop is seen in:

A. Psoriasis of nails
B. Lichen planus of nails
C. Clubbing
D. T. ungium

19. All of the following are staphylococcal lesion *except*:

A. Erysipelas B. Furuncle
C. Impetigo D. Ecthyma

20. Casal's paint necklace is caused by:

A. Lichen planus B. Pellagra
C. Pernicious anemia D. SLE

21. A 5 years old male child has multiple hyperpigmented macules over the trunk. On rubbing the lesion with the rounded end of a pen, he developed urticarial wheal, confined to the border of the lesion. The most likely diagnosis is:

A. Fixed drug eruption
B. Lichen planus
C. Urticaria pigmentosa
D. Urticarial vasculitis

22. After 3 days of fever patient developed maculo erythematous rash lasting for 48 hours diagnosis is:

A. Fifth disease
B. Rubella
C. Measles
D. Roseola infantum

23. Wrong statement is:

A. Mees line in arsenic poisoning
B. Pterygium of nails in lichen planus
C. Onycholysis in psoriasis
D. Koilonychia in megaloblastic anemia (B_{12} def.)

24. Flaky paint appearance of skin is seen in:

A. Dermatitis B. Marasmus
C. Pellagra D. Kwashiorkar

25. A 9 years old boy has multiple itchy erythematosus wheals all over the body for 2 days. There is no respiratory difficulty. Which is the best treatment?

A. Antihelminthics
B. Systemic corticosteroids
C. Antihistamines
D. Adrenaline

26. A 22 years old woman developed small itchy wheals after physical exertion, walking in the sun, eating hot spicy food and when she was angry. The most likely diagnosis is:

A. Chronic idiopathic utricaria
B. Heat urticaria
C. Solar urticaria
D. Cholinergic urticaria

27. A 40 years old farmer with a history of recurrent attacks of porphyria complains of itching when exposes to the sun and maculopapular rash on sun exposed areas, his symptoms are exaggerated in the summer. The diagnosis is:

A. Seborrheic dermatitis
B. Contact dermatitis
C. Psoriasis
D. Porphyria cutanea tarda

28. A 55 years old male, with uncontrolled diabetes mellitus and hypertension, developed severe airborne contact dermatitis. The most appropriate drug for his treatment would be:

A. Systemic corticosteroids
B. Thalidomide
C. Azathioprine
D. Cyclosporine

29. A 45 years old male has multiple grouped vesicular lesions present on the T10 segment dermatome associated with pain. The most likely diagnosis is:

A. Herpes zoster
B. Dermatitis herpetiformis
C. Herpes simplex
D. Scabies

Answers :

1. B	2. A	3. A	4. C,D
5. A	6. A	7. C	8. A
9. C	10. A	11. A	12. C
13. D	14. B	15. A	16. A
17. C	18. A	19. A	20. B
21. C	22. D	23. D	24. D
25. C	26. D	27. D	28. C
29. A			

Section 10

THERAPY

1. Drug of choice for pustular psoriasis:

A. Methotrexate B. Retinoids
C. Mycophenolate mofetil D. Imiquimod

2. Drug of choice for erythrodermic psoriasis:

A. Methotrexate B. Retinoids
C. Mycophenolate mofetil D. Imiquimod

3. Methotrexate causes following:

A. Liver fibrosis
B. Reduced platelet count
C. Hair loss
D. All of the above

4. Which of the following drug is not used as steroid sparing agent?

A. Imiquimod
B. Azathioprine
C. Cyclophosphamide
D. Mycophenolate mofetil

5. Following agent is an example of biologic therapy:

A. Imiquimod
B. Azathioprine
C. Etanercept
D. Mycophenolate mofetil

6. Imiquimod is used in treatment of:

A. Warts B. Acne
C. Psoriasis D. Atopic dermatitis

7. Tacrolimus is used in treatment of:

A. Atopic dermatitis B. Vitiligo
C. Psoriasis D. All of the above

8. Which of the following topical agents is used in psoriasis?

A. Adapalene (0.1%) gel
B. Tazarotene (0.05-0.01%)
C. Tretinoin
D. Isotretinoin

9. One finger tip unit has how many grams of cream?

A. 0.5 gm B. 10 gm
C. 15 gm D. 20 gm

10. Toxic epidermonercrolysis is caused by:

A. Phenytoin B. Pencillin
C. Erythromycin D. Gold

11. Photosensitive lichenoid drug eruption is seen in .... therapy.

A. Rifampicin B. Tetracycline (old)
C. Gold D. Streptomycin

12. Chloroquine cause exacerbation of:

A. Malaria B. Psoriasis
C. DLE D. Photosensitivity

13. SLE like syndrome may be produced by all *except:*

A. Penicillin B. Psoralen
C. Dapsone D. Clofazimine
E. Chlorthiazide

14. A 27 years old sexually active male develops a vesiculobullous lesion on the glans soon after taking tablet paracetamol for fever. The lesion healed with hyperpigmentation. The most likely diagnosis is:

A. Behcet's syndrome
B. Herpes genitalis
C. Fixed drug eruption
D. Pemphigus vulgaris

15. Regarding erythema multiforme all are true *except*:

A. No vesicles
B. Target lesions are seen
C. Involves face and neck regions
D. Sign of internal malignancy

Answers :

1. B	2. A	3. D	4. A
5. C	6. A	7. D	8. B
9. A	10. A, B	11. B	12. B
13. E	14. C	15. D	

Part IV

Controversial MCQs (PGI, AIIMS, AIPG)

Controversial or Wrongly Answered MCQs in Various Guides

The biggest tragedy is that almost *all the guide books* are written by *non dermatologists* with inaccurate answers which are repeated every year in the books. Also except for one book Comprehensive Textbook of Dermatology, *Garg, Sardana* no other book has been written for MCQs.

Here we attempt to answer the wrongly answered MCQ in various guide books. As you would notice most of the Q are sent by students across India and thus the informal format…

1. **Reiter's is commonly caused by…….Some guide books have given the answer as Chlamydia which is a wrong answer.**

Postinfectious or Reactive Arthritis

Reiter's syndrome, a reactive polyarthritis, develops several weeks after ~1% of cases of non-gonococcal urethritis and 2% of enteric infections, particularly those due to **Yersinia enterocolitica, Shigella flexneri,** *Campylobacter jejuni* and *Salmonella* species. Only a minority of these patients have the other findings of classic Reiter's syndrome, including urethritis, conjunctivitis, uveitis, oral ulcers, and rash. Reiter's syndrome is most common among young men (except after *Yersinia* infection) and has been linked to the HLA-B27 locus as a potential genetic predisposing factor.

Patients report *painful, asymmetric oligoarthritis* affecting mainly the **knees, ankles and feet.** Low-back pain is common, and radiographic evidence of sacroiliitis is found in patients with long-standing disease. Most patients recover within 6 months, but prolonged recurrent disease is more common in cases following chlamydial urethritis. Anti-inflammatory agents help to relieve symptoms, but the role of prolonged antibiotic therapy in eliminating microbial antigen from the synovium is controversial.

2. **Treponema can be seen in the CSF in which stage of syphilis?**

   A. Primary syphilis

   B. Secondary syphilis

   C. CNS syphilis

   D. Congenital syphilis

The Answer is B: As because of spirochaetemia the treponema reach the CSF without necessarily causing symptoms. The CNS stage is actually because of an immune reaction to the treponema and at this stage the VDRL may be positive but treponema are not seen. Abnormalities in the CSF have been noted in 13% of patients with untreated primary syphilis, and 25–40% of patients with untreated secondary syphilis. **T. pallidum has been recovered by CSF inoculation into rabbits from upto 30% of patients with primary or secondary syphilis but rarely from those with latent syphilis**. Another study has found that T. pallidum has been demonstrated by animal inoculation or PCR in the CSF of 15–40% of patients with untreated primary and secondary syphilis, even in the absence of other abnormalities. After the initial spirochetal invasion of the CNS during early syphilis, untreated infection may resolve spontaneously, persist as asymptomatic syphilitic meningitis, or progress to symptomatic acute syphilitic meningitis.

Evaluation for Neurosyphilis

Diagnosis

1. **Pleocytosis (>5 white blood cells/mm^3).**
2. Increased protein concentration (>45 mg/dL).
3. VDRL reactivity. CSF abnormalities can be demonstrated in upto **40%** of cases of primary or secondary syphilis and in **25%** of cases of latent syphilis.

T. pallidum has been recovered by CSF inoculation into rabbits from upto **30%** of patients with primary or secondary syphilis but rarely from those with latent syphilis. The presence of *T. pallidum* in CSF is often associated with other CSF abnormalities; however, organisms can be recovered from patients with otherwise normal CSF. Before the advent of penicillin, the risk of developing clinical neurosyphilis was roughly proportional to the intensity of CSF changes.

CSF examination is recommended by the Centers for Disease Control and Prevention (CDC) in the evaluation of ***any seropositive patient*** with neurologic or ophthalmic signs and symptoms, patients with **other late syphilis**, cases of suspected **treatment failure**, and HIV-infected patients with untreated late latent syphilis or syphilis of unknown duration.

The possibility of *asymptomatic neurosyphilis* in some patients with early disease is not addressed by these recommendations. Because standard therapy with penicillin G benzathine fails to result in treponemicidal drug levels in the CSF, some experts also advise lumbar puncture in early syphilis, particularly in patients with HIV infection or if the nontreponemal test titers of> ***1:32***.

The CSF VDRL test is highly specific but is insensitive and may be non-reactive even in cases of symptomatic neurosyphilis. The degree of sensitivity is ***highest in meningovascular and paresis*** and is lower in asymptomatic neurosyphilis and tabes dorsalis. The unabsorbed FTA test on CSF is reactive far more often than the CSF VDRL test in all stages of, but FTA reactivity may reflect passive transfer of serum antibody into the CSF. A non-reactive CSF FTA test, however, may be used to rule out neurosyphilis.

Some Important Facts About the Tests for Syphilis

DG

It is the *most specific* test and is used for both primary stage and secondary syphilis. Darkfield examination has no place in diagnosing late syphilis.

Culture

No method has been developed for culture outside of animals, despite years of trying by many investigators. T. pallidum can be grown in animals, and isolation in rabbits has been used in test of clinical materials.

Serological Tests

FTA-ABS: This test *was highly specific* for T. pallidum and very sensitive but required a fluorescent microscope and highly trained personnel. It has largely been replaced by a card assay that uses hemagglutination as the endpoint (MHA-TP or TPHA). A variation on this test now widely used is the T. pallidum particle agglutination test. These tests are reported without titration, and the result is positive or negative.

TPHA

This is a specific test but it is more useful when it is negative. It is conventionally used to confirm a VDRL test. But the MHA-TP may remain from a prior syphilitic infection, and the genital lesion may be due to another organism altogether, e.g., H. ducreyi. The same may apply even if both tests (VDRL and TPHA) are positive. This is why the search for treponemes by Darkfield examination should be undertaken whenever possible, even though it is time consuming and requires trained personnel, and why tests should be routinely done for other causes of genital ulcer.

A high-titered MHA-TP in the presence of a skin rash strongly supports a diagnosis of secondary syphilis. Nevertheless, the most reliable use of the MHA-TP test is to use *a negative result to exclude the diagnosis of anything other than the earliest stage of primary syphilitic infection.*

STAGE WISE USE OF TESTS

In Primary Syphilis

RPR is positive in about 80% of patients at the time they come to medical attention, often at a relatively low level (< 1:16). The MHA-TP is positive in about 90% of such patients.

In Secondary Syphilis

The RPR is *always positive* and at titers >1:16, as is the MHA-TP.

A negative MHA-TP excludes the diagnosis of syphilis in a patient with a rash that might be secondary infection (so does a negative or low-titer RPR, although the prozone phenomenon rarely may give a false-negative reaction).

In Neurosyphilis

The RPR *rises in some,* but not all forms.

A negative MHA-TP excludes the possibility that neurologic or cardiovascular disease may be syphilitic.

In CVS

The RPR may also be positive at only a low level in cardiovascular syphilis, because weakening of the aortic wall may continue after active disease has burned itself out.

A negative MHA-TP excludes the possibility that neurologic or cardiovascular disease may be syphilitic.

In Gummatous Disease

The RPR is positive at a high level, as might be expected from the immunologic nature of the reaction.

References:

- Harrison Textbook of Medicine, 17th edition.
- Sexually Transmitted Disease by Holmes, 4th edition.

3. **Genodermal disease that can cause skin malignancy are: (December 2003) PGI–Chandigarh**

   A. Xeroderma pigmentosa

   B. Neurofibromatosis

   C. Actinic keratosis

   D. Porphyrea cutanea tarda

The genodermatoses are genetic defect induced skin disorders and here the Ans. is A, B. It should be noted that all the conditions mentioned can cause cancer.

4. **Secondary syphilis is manifested by: (December 2003)**

   A. Painless lymphadenopathy

   B. Pruritic rash

   C. Mucosal erosion

   D. Asymptomatic rash

   E. Mostly asymptomatic

The rash of S2 is non itchy, and has LN with oral mucosal erosions called mucus patch.

Ans. A,C,D,E

5. **Hypo-depigmented lesion is seen in: (June 2004)**
   A. Nevus ito
   B. Nevus depigmentosa
   C. Nevus ota
   D. Nevus anemicus
   E. Freckles

Ans. In guide book is B but it ideally should be both A and D. N anemicus is a pharmacological nevus and presents as a white patch. Ideally though *none of the lesions mentioned are* depigmented .Only vitiligo and albinism are depigmented.

6. **DOC for type 2 reaction leprosy. Thalidomide or steroids.**

This is another controversy that has its origins in guide books. It should be emphasized that the ideal drug is thalidomide as it inhibits TNF alpha which is the main cytokine involved in leprosy. Thus for ENL it is the best drug. Steroids can also be given but we give it in India more often *only because it is cheaper not because it is ideal.*

TYPE 2 LEPRA REACTIONS

This debilitating and chronic reaction is seen most commonly in BL, LL patients. In most cases the onset is after 6 months of therapy or rarely they may occur de novo.

It is a type 3 or immune complex mediated Lepra reaction

Clinical Features

- The classic lesions are tender, erythematous, evanescent nodules referred to as erythema nodosum leprosum (ENL). The systemic involvement manifests in the form of conjunctivitis, keratitis, iritis, iridocyclitis, or chitis, hepatomegaly and lymphadenopathy.

Types

Three patterns of ENL have been described and the acute, multiple and chronic types accounted for 32% and 62% of the cases respectively.

- ***Acute single episode*** is defined as a single episode responding to steroid treatment and this accounts for only 6% of episodes.
- ***Acute multiple ENL:*** This is constituted by recurrent episodes with intervening periods where no treatment is rqeuired.
- ***Chronic ENL:*** In this, the patient needs steroid treatment for more than 6 months and is the most distressing type for the patient and the clinician.

Grading of Reaction

The older classification divides ENL into mild, moderate and severe varieties, but the latest recommendations grades them in two types:

1. A **mild reaction** is one that occurs in the skin only *(as long as it does not occur over a major nerve or in the face*); there may be mild fever and slight swelling (edema) of the limbs.
2. **Severe reactions** affect the nerves or eyes in addition to the skin and the signs include:
   - Pain or tenderness in the nerves.
   - New loss of sensation.
   - New muscle weakness.
   - Reaction in a skin lesion lying over a major nerve.
   - Reaction in a skin lesion on the face.
   - Signs of inflammation in the eye.
   - Severe oedema (swelling) of the limbs.
   - Involvement of other organs, such as testes, lymph nodes or joints.
   - Ulceration of skin lesions.

Therapy

There are broadly, two different approaches to therapy in ENL. The first is a simplistic approach suggested by WHO /ILEP and the second approach is a more flexible approach followed by tertiary care specialists. It should be emphasized that the fixed dose duration approach is usually inadequate and long term steroids may be required. Thus, wherever possible, a suitable adjuvant should be considered.

Box 1: Salient points regarding WHO therapy

In following the WHO guidelines, the understated points should be adhered to:

- If the MDT treatment is already completed, there is no need to restart MDT.
- The total duration of a standard course of corticosteroids (prednisolone) is 12 weeks.
- The total duration of treatment with high dosage of clofazimine should not exceed 12 months. It takes about 4-6 weeks for clofazimine to take full effect in controlling ENL.
- Another drug that is useful in ENL is pentoxifylline, alone or in combination with clofazimine/prednisolone.
- For the reason of its well-known teratogenic side effects, WHO does not support use of thalidomide for the management of ENL in leprosy.

Management in Tertiary Centres

A summary of a suggested regimen is given below which could be followed by specialists in tertiary centres.

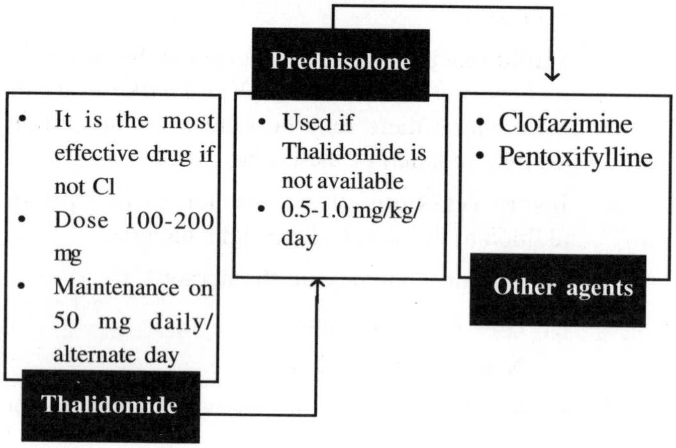

* *The duration of therapy depends on the type of ENL but can continue for upto 12 months.*

Thalidomide: Though this drug is reserved for severe, recalcitrant cases, it is the *most effective and safe drug for ENL.* The cost and the lack of free availability is the major deterrent. The therapy depends largely on the previous exposure to steroids.

Dose Regimen

- *Steroid Naive Patient*—In ENL, thalidomide is dramatically effective in the majority of patients with a response which occurs *within 48 hours*. The starting dose is *100 to 200 mg at night, which can be increased to 100 mg, 3-4 times a day*. Tapering the dose of thalidomide should be started when there is 90% diminution of systemic symptoms or skin lesions. The tapering should be ideally completed in 4 weeks. In case of chronic ENL, a maintenance dose of 100 mg is required. In case of partial effect, prednisone can be added (0.5 to 1.0 mg/kg) and after control has been achieved, prednisone can be tapered over the subsequent 6 to 8 weeks. Another option is to increase the dose of thalidomide to a maximum of 600 mg at bedtime.
- *Patients on Steroids*—A patient already on steroids may have ENL that is *more difficult to control*. It may take several weeks to reduce the dose of steroids and obtain control with thalidomide alone. Thus, first the steroid should be tapered till there is a flare of ENL, at which time thalidomide is initiated at a dose of 100 mg, 4 times a day. It should be noted that thaidomide failure can occur specially in BB, BL cases in which concomitant steroids are invariably needed.

A summary of salient points regarding thalidomide are given below:

Important Points Regarding Thalidomide Use

- The WHO Expert Committee advises that thalidomide should only be given to *men or post-menopausal women who are dependent on corticosteroids.*
- **The ILEP technical bulletin acknowledges the effectiveness of thalidomide and states that 'it has fewer adverse effects than corticosteroids'.**
- Only one month's supply of thalidomide should be prescribed to ensure that regular assessments can be conducted and pregnancy tests are negative before further drugs are dispensed.
- There is little good data concerning the effect of thalidomide on the neural and ocular manifestations of enl which are disabling and occur commonly.
- The patient should be stabilised on the lowest dose of thalidomide that controls the disease and this dose should be continued for a period of 2-3 months.

Books/Reviews

1. Ridley Jopling: Hand Book of Leprosy, 2004.
2. Hastings: Textbook of Leprosy, 1998.
3. Walker SL, Lockwood DN: Leprosy, Clin Dermatol, 2007 Mar-Apr 25(2):165-72.
4. WJ Britton, Diana NJ Lockwood: Leprosy, The Lancet 2004;363:1209-1219.
5. How to Diagnose and Treat Leprosy ILEP.
6. How to Recognize and Manage Leprosy Reactions ILEP.
7. Report of the Eighth Meeting of the WHO Technical Advisory Group on Leprosy Control Aberdeen, Scotland 21st April 2006,WHO.
8. Global Strategy for Further Reducing the Leprosy Burden and Sustaining Leprosy Control Activities 2006-2010 Operational Guidelines.
9. Training manual for medical officers. National Leprosy Eradication Programme Directorate General of Health Services Ministry of Health and Family Welfare, Nirman Bhawan, New Delhi.

7. Vitropressin (in relation to sarcoidosis).

This is same as diascopy and is used for sarcoidosis, lupus vulgaris, granuloma annulare and for diagnosing purpura.

8. Is erythema induratum same as erythema nodosum and thus is EN also a tuberculide.

The only 3 tuberculides are L scrofulosorum papulonecrotic tuberculide and E indurativum and the most common is L scrofulosorum.

9. Most common cause for T. capitis.

In India: T violaceum and M audouinii.

In USA: T tonsurans.

10. What is Majocchi's granuloma?

MAJOCCHI GRANULOMA
- Deep dermatophytic folliculitis, with foreign-body granuloma occurring in response to dermatophytes in the dermis.
- Etiology: Most commonly *T. rubrum*, *T. tonsurans*
- Risk factors
  - Topical glucocorticoid application
  - Systemic immunocompromise
    - Atopic dermatitis
    - Chemotherapy for leukemia, lymphoma
    - Autoimmune disease
    - Solid-organ transplant recipient
- Pathogenesis: Foreign-body response to keratin
- Clinical findings:
  - Types
    - Follicular type with local immunosuppression (topical glucocorticoid use)
    - Subcutaneous nodular type with systemic immunocompromise. Solitary or multiple
  - Folliculocentric papules and pustules arise within an area of epidermal dermatophytosis such as tinea incognito.
  - Distribution: Any hair-bearing area; scalp, face, forearms, dorsum of hands/feet, shaved legs.

Synonym: Dermatophytic or trichophytic granuloma.

It is an infection caused by dermatophytes and is described under T corporis.

11. Most common veneral disease gonorrohea LGV?

The most common STD is urethritis the most common type is NGU and it is caused by C trachomatis. Also the most common GUD is herpes genitalis.

12. Primary skin lesions are seen in all *except*:

A. Bowen's disease

B. Reiter's disease

C. Psoriasis

D. Lichen planus

Most guide books have the *right answer but the wrong explanation*. It is Reiters as it has *Secondary Skin Lesions* (Keratoderma blenorrhagicum and circinate balanitis) and not the primary lesions like papules (LP) plaques (Psoriasis and Bowen's disease).

13. A child comes with itchy papules on the forehead face and limbs which worsen in rainy season and improve in winters. What is the most likely diagnosis?

A. Photoallergic dermatoses

B. Atopic dermatoses

C. Solar urticaria

D. Insect bite reaction

A.	• Sunlight induced, exposed site, usually adults
B.	• Eczema, asthma, worsens in winters
C.	• Sunlight, wheals, adults
D.	• Child, summers, rains, mosquito bites*

* *Adults do not have a reaction to insect bites as they have acquired a immunity to it.*

14. A female is put on isotretinoin she decides to stop the medicine after how much time can she conceive?

A. 2 months B. 3 months

C. 3 years D. 1 year

Ans. B

15. Thimble pitting is seen in:

A. Alopecia areata B. Psoriasis

C. L planus D. T unguium

This Q has been wrongly answered because a UG book of skin has given the wrong answer in the book.

Thimble pits refers to the fine pits seen in (A) alopecia areata NOT PSORIASIS.

16. Treponema pallidum can be found in CSF in:

A. Primary syphilis B. Secondary syphilis

C. Tertiary syphilis D. Tabes dorsalis

The answer is B the reason is that the treponema dissemiante all over in the secondary stage and about 30% of S2 case have treponema in the CSF. In fact 40% of these cases also have CSF abnormalities. Interestingly in tertiary stage the problem is because of the CMI and the treponema are sparse.

17. DIF is negative in: (PGI 2010)

A. Hailey hailey disease B. Darier disease

C. Bullous pemphigoid D. Herpes gestationalis

A very simple of answering this is that which condition is not autoimmune in that the DIF will be negative.

A.	• It is a non-immune condition also called benign familial pemphigus
B.	• It is a genetic disorder with seborrheic sites involved with papules that are greasy
C.	• Linear IgG and C3 on BMZ (D/F)
D.	• C3 (D/F)

18. A 10-year-old school girl has recurrent episodes of boils on the scalp.The boils subsided with antibiotics but recur after some time. The most likely cause of recurrence is:

A. Primary immunodeficiency syndrome

B. Pediculis capitis

It is important to note that even P capitis can present with recurrent boils, so if the Q has itching with boils the answer is P capitis otherwise the answer is A.

19. Treatment of acute neuritis in lepra 1 reaction is all *except*:

A. Dapsone B. Corticosteroid

C. Thalidomide D. I and D

Yes the answer to this question is (C) thalidomide, this is because thalidomide does not prevent neuritis as it works on TNF alpha.

20. Underlying internal malignancy is NOT shown by:

A. Acanthosis nigrans

B. Bullous pyoderma

C. Granuloma annulare

D. Erythema gyratum repens

Answer is (B) Pyoderma is a bacterial infection seen in children and malignancy is not seen commonly with it. There is another condition called bullous pyoderma gangrenosum which is associated with malignancy.

21. There is an unnecessary controversy between (a) atopic dermatitis (b) infant eczematoid dermatitis.

There is a entity called **Infantile AD** which is the first phase of AD where lesions are seen on the extensors but the term *infant eczematoid dermatitis is INCORRECT*. There is no such term Dermatology. It is a crude term to describe any eczema occurring in infants.

There is another term called *Infected eczematoid dermatitis* and *infectious eczematoid dermatitis* which are different as in the first an eczema gets infected while in the second the infection cause eczema.

AD

Age of Onset: First 2 months of life and by the first years in 60% of patients. 30% are seen for the first time by age 5, and only 10% develop AD between 6 and 20 years of age. Rarely AD has an adult onset.

Eliciting Factors: Inhalants, Microbial Agents (Exotoxins of Staphylococcus aureus), Autoallergens and Foods (eggs, milk, peanuts, soybeans, fish and wheat).

Other Exacerbating Factors: Skin Barrier Disruption (decrease of barrier function associated with impaired filaggrin production, reduced ceramide levels, and increased transepidermal water loss). Infections (S. aureus; group A streptococcus; rarely fungus), season (improves in summer, flares in winter), clothing (wool is an important trigger) and emotional stress.

Infantile AD: The lesions present as red skin,tiny vesicles on "puffy" surface. Scaling, exudation with wet crusts and cracks (fissures), skin lesions seem to be a reaction to itching and rubbing.

Childhood-type AD: The lesions are papular, lichenified plaques, erosions, crusts, especially on the antecubital and popliteal fossae the neck and face; may be generalized.

Adult-type AD: There is a similar distribution, mostly flexural but also face and neck, with lichenification and excoriations being the most conspicuous symptoms.

DIAGNOSIS

History in infancy, clinical findings (typical distribution sites, morphology of lesions, white dermatographism).

Therapy

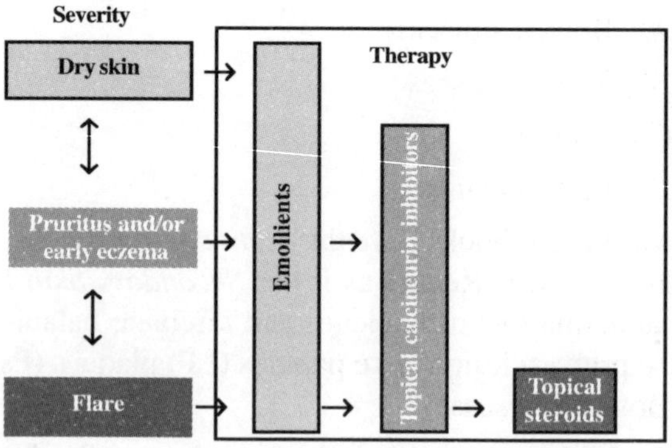

OTHER QUESTIONS

1. Normal turnover time of skin is:

A. 2 weeks

B. 4 weeks

C. 6 weeks

D. 8 weeks

(The correct answer is about 52-75 days that roughly corresponds to 8 weeks.)

2. **A child presents with a solitary white well defined macule on his right thigh, diagnosis is:**

A. Piebaldism

B. Albinism

C. Nevus achromicus

D. Acral vitiligo

(This is same as nevus depigmentosus. But another possibility is segmental vitiligo and if it is blanchable, nevus anemicus.)

3. **Minor clinical features in atopic dermatitis all *except*:**

A. Dry skin

B. Pruritus

C. Morgan fold

D. Pityriasis alba

E. Dermatographism

(Actually the Q is wrongly framed it should be all except as the only 4 major features are:

- Pruritus.
- Chronic relapsing course.
- Typical distribution.
- Personal or family history.)

4. **Kaposi varicelliform eruption is seen in:**

A. Atopic dermatitis

B. Darier's disease

C. Lichen planus

D. Varicella zoster

(KVE is caused by *HSV-1, HSV-2, coxsackievirus A16, or vaccinia virus* infecting a preexisting dermatosis.

- Most commonly, it is caused by a disseminated HSV infection in patients with **atopic dermatitis.** For this reason, it is also referred to as eczema herpeticum.
- KVE has also been associated with *mycosis fungoides, pityriasis rubra pilaris, neurodermatitis, irritant contact dermatitis, congenital ichthyosiform erythroderma, ichthyosis vulgaris, pemphigus foliaceus, benign familial pemphigus (Hailey-Hailey disease),* ***Darier's disease****, Wiskott-Aldrich syndrome, Sézary syndrome, seborrheic dermatitis, skin grafts, burns, cowpox and rosacea.)*

5. **A 22 years old woman developed small wheals after physical exertion walking in the sun, eating hot spicy food and when she was angry, the most likely cause is:**

A. Chronic idiopathic urticaria

B. Heat urticaria

C. Solar urticaria

D. Cholinergic urticaria

(Though the answer is cholinergic urticaria if they only mention sunlight then the most likely answer is solar urticaria.)

6. **All may lead to hives and wheals *except:***

A. Cold

B. Hepatitis C

C. Serum sickness

D. Typhoid fever

(In this all can cause urticaria but statistically speaking the least common is typhoid.)

Immunologic Causes

Type I IgE-mediated

Foods: Tree nuts, legumes, crustacea, mollusks, fish, eggs, milk, soy, wheat.

Organic substances: Preservatives, latex, hymenoptera venom.

Medications: Penicillin, cephalosporin, aspirin, NSAIDs.

Aeroallergens: Dust mites, pollens, molds, animal dander.

Type II cytoxic antibody-mediated: Transfusion reaction.

Type III antigen-antibody mediated: **Serum sickness reaction.**

Type IV delayed hypersensitivity: Medication, food handling, or exposure to animals.

Autoimmune disease: Hashimoto's disease, systemic lupus erythematosus, vasculitis, hepatitis.

Infection: Viral (e.g., cytomegalovirus, Epstein-Barr, **hepatitis**), parasitic, fungal or bacterial.

Nonimmunologic Causes

Physical stimuli: Exposure to sun, water or **temperature extremes;** delayed pressure (e.g., wearing a heavy backpack); vibration.

Direct mast cell degranulation: Opiates, vancomycin (vancocin), aspirin, radiocontrast media, dextran, muscle relaxants, bile salts, NSAIDs.

Foods containing high levels of histamines: Strawberries, tomatoes, shrimp, lobster, cheese, spinach, eggplant.

7. All are true regarding hereditary angioedema *except:*

A. Dysfunction of the enzyme is the most common cause

B. Enzyme is C1-INH

C. C1 inhibitor targets Hageman factor

D. Complement C_4 and C_2 decrease

E. Bradykinin level decrease during attack

This question is particularly interesting and on analyzing the extract below the last is wrong. The points in italics will help in questions of angioedema.

Angioedema Hereditary: Increased susceptibility to angioedema can result from either an *inherited defect in C1-esterase inhibitor* (C1-INH) activity or an *acquired deficiency of C1-INH*. The inherited form of the disease, known as hereditary angioedema, is rare. There are two principal types of hereditary angioedema: *type 1*, which accounts for 80% to 85% of cases and is caused by decreased production of C1-INH, and *type 2*, in which normal or elevated amounts of functionally deficient C1-INH are produced. *A third*, very rare form of hereditary angioedema that may be X-linked has recently been described in women.

Acquired angioedema results from increased metabolism or destruction of C1-INH. Two types of acquired angioedema have been described.

Type 1, which is caused by excessive activation of complement and subsequent consumption of C1-INH, typically occurs in patients with *rheumatologic disorders and B cell lymphoproliferative diseases*. Patients with *type 2* produce autoantibodies against C1-INH, leading to its inactivation.

Bradykinin and leukotrienes are increased during the attacks.

Clinical Features

IgE-induced angioedema are most likely to present with *concomitant urticaria*. This form of angioedema may be pruritic and may progress to an anaphylactic reaction.

ACE inhibitors is nonpruritic and rarely occurs with urticaria. No sex predominance has been noted in patients without gastrointestinal tract involvement, but all patients with GI involvement have been women.

Complement-activated angioedema is never pruritic and is *not accompanied by urticaria*. In **20% to 25%** of patients with hereditary angioedema, there is *no family history* of the disease (these cases may represent new mutations). Therefore, a *positive family history of hereditary angioedema is not a prerequisite* for the consideration of this disorder in the differential diagnosis when typical symptoms are present. Symptoms of hereditary angioedema are usually mild or nonexistent during childhood, typically first manifesting during the second decade of life. Acquired angioedema usually develops during or after the fourth decade of life.

Laboratory Tests

IgE-induced drug reactions are readily identifiable with skin-prick tests or RAST.

In complement-activated angioedema, a *low level of the complement component C4* is a constant finding and therefore represents a sensitive screening test. A normal level, especially during an attack, rules out both hereditary and acquired angioedema. In patients with suspected complement-activated angioedema, confirmation of the diagnosis can be obtained by measuring antigenic levels of C1-INH, which are low. In 85% of patients, or functional levels, which are low in 100% of patients.

Hereditary forms of complement-activated angioedema can be distinguished from acquired forms by measurement of *C1q complement*—levels of which are normal in hereditary.

8. A 9 years old has multiple itchy wheals all over the body with no respiratory difficulty. What is the best treatment?

A. Antihelminthics

B. Corticosteroids

C. Antihistaminics

D. Adrenaline

(In children worms are a common cause of urticaria and in the absence of angioedema and dyspnoea adrenaline has no role.)

9. A patient with psoriasis was started on systemic steroids. After stopping the treatment the patient developed universally red plaques losing their margin all over the body, what is the most likely diagnosis?

A. Drug induced reaction

B. Pustular psoriasis

C. Bacterial infection

D. Erythrodermic psoriasis

(> 80 % BSA involvement is seen in erythroderma. Sudden stopping of steroid leads to pustular psoriasis, so if the same Q has the line *pustules develop all over the body* the answer is B.)

10. The only indication of giving steroid in pustular psoriasis is:

A. Psoriatic erythroderma in pregnancy

B. Psoriatic in a patient with cirrhosis

C. Moderate arthritis

D. Extensive lesions

(Most books wrongly give the answer as extensive lesions. The only indication of monotherapy with steroids is in pregnancy.)

11. Use of PUVA:

A. Pigmented purpuric dermatoses

B. Herpes zoster

C. MF

D. Lupus panniculitis

E. Lichenoid dermatitis of gougerot and blum

12. PUVA therapy is used for:

A. Psoriasis

B. Lichen planus

C. Freckles

D. Lentigines

E. Melasma

(The most common indications are severe psoriasis, vitiligo, localized pustular psoriasis, cutaneous T-cell lymphoma, lichen planus, atopic dermatitis. Rarely used for pigmented purpuric dermatosis.)

13. Which layer of skin causes vesicular change in case of burns?

A. Basal layer

B. Papillary layer

C. Epidermis

D. Dermis

(Vesicular changes are because of changes in the papillary dermis.)

14. Morbilliform eruption is seen in all *except*:

A. Scarlet fever

B. Rubella

C. TSS

D. Measles

E. Mumps

- "Morbilliform" refers to a resemblance to the rash of measles (morbilli is Latin for measles); measles is a rare disease now, but morbilliform eruptions are common.
- Amorbilliform eruption is symmetrically distributed on the trunk and proximal extremities, and consists of bright pink macules and slightly raised papules ("maculopapular").
- Causes range from measles, rubella, drug eruption to Scarlet fever, erythema infectiosum, kawasaki, roseola, serum sickness, infectious mononucleosis.

15. Acantholytic cells in pemphigus are derived from:

A. S granulosum

B. S spinosum

C. S basale

D. LC cell

(The acantholytic cells are derived from the destruction of desmosome and the layers affected in P vulgaris are primarily the S basale and spinosum which has more layers than S basale.

The best answer is S spinosum. In fact S basale is not destroyed as the hemidesmosome which attach it to the dermis are intact.)

(Histopathology demonstrates an *intradermal* blister. The earliest changes consist of intercellular edema with loss of intercellular attachments in the basal layer. *Suprabasal* epidermal cells separate from the basal cells to form clefts and blisters. Basal cells are separated from one another and stand like a *row of tombstones* on the floor of the blister, **but they remain attached to the basement membrane**. Blister cells contain some acantholytic cells. Histopathology can help differentiate PV from pemphigus foliaceous, which demonstrates a more superficial epidermal cleavage.

PV antigen: Intercellular adhesion in the epidermis involves several keratinocyte cell surface molecules. Pemphigus antibody binds to keratinocyte cell surface molecules ***desmoglein 1*** and ***desmoglein 3***. The binding of antibody to desmoglein may have a direct effect on desmosomal adherens or may trigger a cellular process that results in acantholysis.

Tzanck preparation is a smear taken from the base of a blister or an oral erosion that contains acantholytic cells. Blistering is preceded by *eosinophilic spongiosis* in some patients. The superficial dermis has a mild, superficial, mixed inflammatory infiltrate, which includes some eosinophils.)

16. An autoimmune disease is all *except*:

A. Psoriasis

B. Pemphigus

C. Lichen planus

D. Acne vulgaris

17. Genetic predisposition is seen in which disease?

A. Lichen planus

B. Bullous pemphigoid

C. Pemphigus vulgaris

D. Epidermolysis bullosa

18. Genodermal disease that can cause skin malignancy are:

A. Xeroderma pigmentosa

B. Neurofibromatosis

C. Actinic keratosis

D. PCT

19. Following are signs of internal malignancy *except:*

A. Tuberous sclerosis

B. Acanthosis nigricans

C. Clubbing

D. Dermatomyositis

(Curth proposed the following criteria to define a paraneoplastic syndrome:

- The malignancy and syndrome must appear at the same time, and their clinical courses should not significantly differ.
- Remote cutaneous manifestations should be specific to the tumor causing them.
- Paraneoplastic syndromes should be uncommon relative to the prevalence of the cancer.
- The paraneoplastic syndrome and the cancer should be demonstrably associated (**papulosquamous disorders),** tripe palms, acrokeratosis paraneoplastica, Bazex syndrome, ***acanthosis nigricans***, acquired ichthyosis, pityriasis rotunda, sign of Leser-Trelat, extramammary Paget's disease, florid cutaneous papillomatosis, palmoplantar keratoderma, **erythematous lesions,** necrolytic migratory erythema, erythema gyratum repens, Sweet syndrome, hypertrophic osteoarthropathy multicentric reticulohistiocytosis, dermatomyositis, bullous lesions, paraneoplastic pemphigus, hypertrichosis lanuginosa acquisita, Trousseau syndrome, carcinoid tumors.)

20. An 8 years old male from Bihar presents with a 6 months history of ill defined hypopigmented slightly atrophic macule on the face. The most likely diagnosis is:

A. Pityriasis alba

B. Indeterminate leprosy

C. Morphoea

D. Calcium deficiency

(If the questions does not have Bihar then the answer is morphoea.)

21. Manifestations of ENL include all *except:*

A. Pancreatitis

B. Fever

C. Hepatitis

D. Arthiritis

E. Cutaneous nodules

(It is one of the uncommon orgams involved but the only organs not involved is ovary, CNS and uterus.)

22. A 45-year-old male had multiple hypoaesthetic erythematous large plaques with elevated margins on trunk and extremities. His ulnar nerve and lateral popliteal nerve on both sides was enlarged. The diagnsosis is:

A. LL

B. BT

C. BB

D. BL

(Plaques are seen in TT, BT and BB.

BL and LL have in addition macules and papules.

In BB there are features of TT and LL that is plaques, macules and papules.

Multiple nerve enlarged is seen in BT, BB, BL, LL.

So in this Q the best answer is BT.)

23. Best method of treatment of ulnar nerve abscess in case of leprosy is:

A. High dose of steroid

B. Incision and drainage

C. Halidomide

D. Clofazimine

- (Nerve decompression is used when signs of entrapment have not cleared after 3-4 weeks of steroid therapy, when function deteriorates despite steroid therapy, or when signs of nerve abscess or chronic entrapment are evident.
- If you incise a motor nerve there will be iatrogenic palsy and nerve abscess are usually de to reaction and they respond dramatically to steroid.)

  Denom: The only abscess **not** drained primarily is nerve abscess.

24. Skin smear is negative in:

A. Indeterminate leprosy B. Neuritic lesion
C. Lepromatous D. Borderline

(Always negative in neuritic rarely positive in indeterminate.)

25. In leprosy which of the following is not seen?

A. Abnormal EMG
B. Voluntary muscle wasting
C. Decreased proprioception
D. Decreased response to tactile sensation
E. Increased response to tactile sensation

(The earliest feature is hyperpathia so option C is right.)

26. Streptomycin is useful in the treatment of:

A. Granuloma inguinale B. LGV
C. Syphilis D. Chancroid

(For resistant cases gentamicin is given.)

27. True about syphilis is all *except:*

A. VDRL is sensitive
B. Infection leads to lifelong immunity
C. IgM and IgA
D. T pallidum when inoculated in a rabbit produces progressive disease

28. Lymphadenopathy is seen in all *except*:

A. Primary syphilis B. Donovaniosis
C. LGV D. Chancroid

29. Treatment of both partners is recommended in all *except*:

A. Candida B. Gardenella vaginalis
C. Herpes D. Trichomoniasis vaginalis

30. In secondary syphilis all are seen *except:*

A. C lata
B. Interstitial keratitis
C. Arthritis
D. Proteinuria

(All are correct but the last is the rarest.)

Answers :

1. D	**2. C**	**3. B**	**4. A,B**
5. D	**6. D**	**7. E**	**8. A,C**
9. D	**10. A**	**11. A, E**	**12. A,B**
13. B	**14. C**	**15. B**	**16. D**
17. D	**18. A**	**19. A**	**20. B**
21. A	**22. B**	**23. A**	**24. B**
25. C	**26. A**	**27. D**	**28. B**
29. B	**30. D**		

Part V

AIPG, AIIMS MCQs (1990-2009)
PGI, DPG, UPSC (2007-09)

Actual papers of last 12 years

AIPG

1991-2009

AIPG 2009

1. **Primary skin lesions are seen in all *except:***
   A. Bowen's disease B. Reiter's
   C. Psoriasis D. Lichen planus

2. **Scarring alopecia is associated with:**
   A. Alopecia areata B. Tinea capitis
   C. Androgenic alopecia D. Lichen planus

3. **A neonate with focal skin lesions and hypoplastic limbs causative agent:**
   A. Cytomegalovirus
   B. Herpes simplex type 3
   C. Toxoplasma
   D. T. pallidum

4. **Patient present with 5 days fever and raised erythematous lesions. Which on biopsy revealed neutrophilic infiltrate? What is a most probable diagnosis?**
   A. ENL
   B. Sweet syndrome
   C. Erythema nodosum diminuta
   D. EED

5. **Involvement of sweat glands and hair follicles with granuloma around the hair follicles is seen in:**
   A. Lichen scrofulosum
   B. Papulonecrotic tuberculid
   C. Lupus vulgaris
   D. Miliary TB

6. **Acral erythema/red palms is seen with all *except:***
   A. Adriamycin (Doxorubicin)
   B. Cytosine arabinoside
   C. 5-fluorouracil
   D. MMF

7. **In tuberous sclerosis triad all are seen *except:***
   A. Facial angiomatosis
   B. Mental retardation
   C. Seizures
   D. Rhabdomyosarcoma

Answers :

1. B	**2. D**	**3. B**	**4. B**
5. A	**6. D**	**7. D**	

AIPG 2008

1. **Contact allergy associated with:**
   A. Anaphylactoid reactions
   B. IgE mediated reactions
   C. CMI
   D. Type II reaction

2. **Male with patchy loss of scalp hair, eyebrows and beard with grey hair:**
   A. Alopecia areata
   B. Anagen effluvium
   C. Telogen effluvium
   D. Androgenic alopecia

3. **DOC for pregnant woman in 2nd trimester with pustular psoriasis:**
   A. Prednisolone B. Dapsone
   C. Acitretin D. Methotrexate

4. **Female with painful long standing persistent oral lesions with suprabasal acantholysis on biopsy is:**
   A. Pemphigus vulgaris B. Aphthosis
   C. EM D. Bullous pemphigoid

5. **DOC for tertiary syphilis:**
   A. Procaine penicillin
   B. Benzathine penicillin
   C. Crystalline penicillin
   D. Doxycycline

6. **Dharmendra index and Jopling's classification is for:**
   A. TB B. Leprosy
   C. Syphilis D. Leishmaniasis

7. **DOC for lepra II reactions:**
   A. Thalidomide B. Corticosteroids
   C. Clofazimine D. Dapsone

8. **NF-1 associated with:**
   A. Choroidal hemangioma
   B. Glaucoma
   C. Cataract
   D. Rhabdomyomasaicone

9. **Male from West Bengal with hyperkeratosis of palm and soles with transverse nail lines:**
   A. Chronic arsenic poisoning
   B. Pb poisoning

C. Au poisoning
D. Thallium poisoning

10. Immunomodulator for genital warts is:

A. Imiquimod B. Zn
C. Calcium D. Podophyllin

11. Not an antifungal:

A. Caspofungin B. Undecyclinic acid
C. Ciclopirox D. Clofazimine

12. Yaws all true *except:*

A. Is an STD
B. Seen in children
C. Usually seen on trauma prone sites
D. Caused by treponema pertenue

13. All are zoonosis *except:*

A. HIV B. Plague
C. JE D. TB

14. Gumma is seen in:

A. Tertiary stage of syphilis B. Sarcoidosis
C. Tuberculosis D. Leprosy

15. Leucovorin used in psoriasis with:

A. Methotrexate B. Septran
C. Azathioprine D. Retinoids

16. A male comes with painful genital ulcers with history of contact of 5 days, the most likely cause is:

A. Syphilis B. Chancre
C. Herpes D. Chancroid

17. A female patient has abdominal pain followed by purpuric lesions on the lower limb. The most likely diagnosis is:

A. Henoch-Schönlein purpura
B. Leucocytoclastic vasculitis
C. CBDC
D. Dermatitis herpetiformis

Answers :

1. C	2. A	3. A	4. A
5. C	6. B	7. A	8. B
9. A	10. A	11. D	12. A
13. D	14. A	15. A	16. D
17. A			

AIPG 2008

1. A male patient presents with patchy loss of hair on scalp, eyebrows and beard. He also gives history of rapid greying of hair in few areas. Likely diagnosis:

A. Alopecia areata
B. Anagen effluvium
C. Telogen effluvium
D. Androgenetic alopecia

2. A 40 years female developed persistent oral ulcers followed by multiple flaccid bullae on trunk and extremities. Direct examination of a skin biopsy immunofluorescence showed intracellular IgG deposits in the epidermis and suprabasal with acantholyitic cells. The probable diagnosis is:

A. Pemphigus vulgaris
B. Pemphigoid
C. Erythema multiforme
D. Dermatitis herpetiformis

3. A heterosexual male presents with multiple non-indurated painful ulcers with undermined edges and enlarged lymph nodes 5 days after exposure. Most likely diagnosis is:

A. Herpes genitalis B. LGV
C. Primary chancre D. Chancroid

4. Drug of choice for a pregnant woman in 2nd trimester with pustular psoriasis:

A. Prednisolone B. Dapsone
C. Acitretin D. Methotrexate

5. Drug of choice for type 2 lepra reaction:

A. Thalidomide B. Steroids
C. Clofazimine D. Rifampicin

Answers :

1. A	2. A	3. D	4. A
5. A			

AIPG 2006

1. A patient had seven irregular hyperpigmented macules on the trunk and multiple small hyperpigmented macules in axillae and groins since early childhood. There were no other skin lesions. Which is the most likely investigation to support the diagnosis?

A. Slit lamp examination of eye

B. Measurement of intraocular tension
C. Examination of fundus
D. Retinal artery aniography

2. **Pterygium of nail is characteristically seen in:**
A. Lichen planus B. Psoriasis
C. Tinea unguium D. Alopecia areata

3. **A 24 years unmarried woman has multiple nodular cystic putular and comedonic lesions on face, upper back and shoulders for 2 years. Drug of choice for her treatment would be:**
A. Acitretin B. Isotretinoin
C. Doxycycline D. Azithromycin

4. **A 45 years old farmer has itchy erythematous papular lesions on face, neck, area of chest, dorsum of hands and forearms for 3 years. The lesions are more severe in summers and improve by 75% in winters. The most appropriate test to diagnose the condition would be:**
A. Skin biopsy
B. Estimation of IgE levels in blood
C. Patch test
D. Intradermal prick test

5. **A 6 months old infant had itchy erythematous papules and exudative lesions on scalp, face, groins and axillae for 1 month. She also had vesicular lesions on the palms. Most likely diagnosis is:**
A. Congenital syphilis
B. Seborrheic dermatitis
C. Scabies
D. Psoriasis

6. **In which of the following conditions parakeratosis most frequently occurs?**
A. Actinic keratosis
B. Seborrheic keratosis
C. Molluscum contagiosum
D. Basal cell carcinoma

Answers :

1. A	**2. A**	**3. B**	**4. C**
5. C	**6. A**		

AIPG 2005

1. **A 16 years boy presented with asymptomatic multiple erythematous annular lesions with a collarette of scales at the periphery of the lesions present on the trunk. Most likely diagnosis is:**
A. Pityriasis versicolor
B. Pityriasis alba
C. Pityriasis rosea
D. Pityriasis rubra pilaris

2. **All of the following drugs are effective in treatment of pityriasis versicolor *except:***
A. Selenium sulfide B. Ketoconazole
C. Griseofulvin D. Clotrimazole

3. **An 8 years boy from Bihar presents with a 6 months history of an ill-defined hypopigmented slightly atrophic macule on the face. Most likely diagnosis is:**
A. Pityriasis alba
B. Indeterminate leprosy
C. Morphea
D. Calcium deficiency

4. **A 40 years woman presents with a 2 years history of erythematous papulopustular lesions on the convexities of the face. There is a background of erythema and telangiectasia. Most likely diagnosis is:**
A. Acne vulgaris
B. Rosacea
C. SLE
D. Polymorphic light eruption

5. **A 36 years old factory worker developed itchy annular scaly plaques in both the groins. Application of a corticosteroid ointment led to a temporary relief but the plaque continued to extend at the periphery. Most likely diagnosis is:**
A. Erythema annulare centrifugum
B. Granuloma annulare
C. Annular lichen planus
D. Tinea cruris

6. **A 27 years sexually active male develops a vesiculobullous lesion on the glans soon after taking tablet paracetamol for fever. The lesion healed with hyperpigmentation. Most likely diagnosis:**
A. Behcet's syndrome
B. Herpes genitalis
C. Fixed drug eruption
D. Pemphigus vulgaris

7. **The only definite indication for giving systemic corticosteroids in pustular psoriasis is:**
   A. Psoriatic erythroderma with pregnancy
   B. Psoriasis in a patient with alcoholic cirrhosis
   C. Moderate arthritis
   D. Extensive lesions

Answers :

1. C	2. C	3. B	4. B
5. D	6. C	7. A	

AIPG 2004

1. **A 30 years old male had severely itchy papulo-vesicular lesions on extremities, knees, elbows and buttocks for one year. Direct immunofluorescence staining of the lesions showed IgA deposition at dermoepidermal junction. The most probable diagnosis is:**
   A. Pemphigus vulgaris
   B. Bullous pemphigoid
   C. Dermatitis herpetiformis
   D. Nummular eczema

2. **A 5 years old male child has multiple hyper-prigmented macules over the trunk. On rubbing the lesion with the rounded end of a pen, he developed urticarial wheal, confined to the border of the lesion. The most likely diagnosis is:**
   A. Fixed drug eruption
   B. Lichen planus
   C. Urticaria pigmentosa
   D. Urticarial vasculitis

3. **A 25 years old man presents with recurrent episodes of flexural eczema, contact urticaria, recurrent skin infections and severe abdominal cramps and diarrhoea upon taking sea foods. He is suffering from:**
   A. Seborrheic dermatitis
   B. Atopic dermatitis
   C. Airborne contact dermatitis
   D. Nummular dermatitis

Answers :

1. C	2. C	3. B

AIPG 2003

1. **A 40 years old male developed persistent oral ulcers followed by multiple flaccid bullae on trunk and extremities. Direct examination of a skin biopsy immunofluorescence showed intercellular IgG deposits in the epidermis. The most probable diagnosis is:**
   A. Pemphigus vulgaris
   B. Bullous pemphigoid
   C. Bullous lupus erythematosus
   D. Epidermolysis bullosa acquisita

2. **Acantholysis is characteristic of:**
   A. Pemphigus vulgaris
   B. Pemphigoid
   C. Erythema multiforme
   D. Dermatitis herpetiformis

3. **A 5 years boy has multiple asymptomatic oval and circular faintly hypopigmented macules with fine scaling on his face. The most probable clinical diagnosis is:**
   A. Pityriasis versicolor
   B. Indeterminate leprosy
   C. Pityriasis alba
   D. Acrofacial vitiligo

4. **An eleven years old boy is having tinea capitis on his scalp. The most appropriate line of treatment is:**
   A. Oral griseofulvin therapy
   B. Topical griseofulvin therapy
   C. Shaving of the scalp
   D. Selenium sulphide shampoo

5. **The test likely to help in diagnosis of a patient who presents with an itchy annular plaque on the face is:**
   A. Gram's stain
   B. Potassium hydroxide mount
   C. Tissue smear
   D. Wood's lamp examination

6. **An 8-month-old child presented with itchy, exudative lesions on the face, palms and soles. The siblings also have similar complaints. The treatment of choice is such a patient is:**
   A. Systemic ampicillin
   B. Topical betamethasone
   C. Systemic prednisolone
   D. Topical permethrin

7. **The most frequent cause of recurrent genital ulceration in a sexually active male is:**

A. Herpes genitalis B. Aphthous ulcer
C. Syphilis D. Chancroid

8. The syndromic management of urethral discharge includes treatment of:
A. Neisseria gonorrhoeae and herpes genitalis
B. Chlamydia trachomatis and herpes ganitalis
C. Neisseria gonorrhoeae and chlamydia trachomatis
D. Syphilis and chancroid

Answers :

1. A	2. A	3. C	4. A
5. B	6. D	7. A	8. C

AIPG 2002

1. Multiple erythematous annular lesions with peripheral collorette of scales arranged predominantly over trunk are seen in:
A. Pityriasis versicolor
B. Pityriasis rubra
C. Pityriasis rosea
D. Pityriasis lichenoides chronica

2. All of the following are given for the treatment of pityriasis versicolor, *except*:
A. Ketoconazole B. Griseofulvin
C. Clotrimazole D. Selenium sulphide

3. A patient with psoriasis was started on systemic steroids. After stopping treatment, the patient developed generalized pustules all over the body. The cause is most likely to be:
A. Drug induced reaction
B. Pustular psoriasis
C. Bacterial infections
D. Septicemia

4. Wickheim's stria are seen in:
A. Lichen nitidus B. Lichenoid eruption
C. Lichen striatus D. Lichen planus

5. Griseofulvin is given for the treatment of fungal infection in finger nail dermatophytosis for:
A. 4 weeks **B.** 6 weeks
C. 2 months **D.** 3 months

6. After 3 days of fever patient developed maculo erythematous rash that lasted for 48 hours. The most likely diagnosis is:
A. Fifth disease B. Rubella
C. Measles D. Roseola infantum

7. Exfoliative dermatitis can be due to all the following diseases, *except:*
A. Drug hypersensitivity B. Pityriasis rubra
C. Pityriasis rosea D. Psoriasis

8. Genital elephantiasis is caused by:
A. Donovanosis
B. Congenital syphilis
C. Herpes genitalis
D. Lymphogranuloma venerum

Answers :

1. C	2. B	3. B	4. D
5. D	6. D	7. C	8. D

AIPG 2001

1. A man aged 30 years presents with alopecia, boggy scalp swelling and easily pluckable hair. Next step in establishing diagnosis would be:
A. KOH smear B. Culture sensitivity
C. Biopsy D. None of the above

2. Most common organism causing tinea capitis is:
A. Trichophyton tonsurans B. Microsporum
C. Epidermophyton D. Candida albicans

3. A young man aged 19 years develops a painless penile ulcer 9 days after sexual intercourse with a professional sex worker, likely diagnosis is:
A. Chancroid B. Herpes
C. Chancre D. Traumatic ulcer

4. An infant presents with itchy lesions over the groin and prepuce. All of the following are indicated in this patient *except*:††
A. Bathe and apply scabicidal solution
B. Treatment should be extended to all family members
C. Dispose all clothes by burning
D. Start the patient on I.V. antibiotics

5. A boy aged 8 years from Tamilnadu presents with white, non-anesthetic, nonscaly, hypopigmented macule on his face, likely diagnosis is:
A. Pityriasis alba

B. Pityriasis versicolor
C. Indeterminate leprosy
D. Pure neuritic leprosy

6. A 20 years old male patient from Jaipur, presents with an erythematous lesion on the cheek with central crusting, likely diagnosis is:

A. SLE
B. Lupus vulgaris
C. Chilblains
D. Cutaneous leishmaniasis

7. A 19 years aged girl presents with light brown pigmentation over the malar eminences, likely diagnosis is:

A. Chloasma
B. SLE
C. Melasma
D. Melanoma

8. A girl, aged 19 presents with arthritis and a photosensitive rash on the cheek, likely diagnosis is:

A. SLE
B. Chloasma
C. Stevens-Johnson syndrome
D. Lymes disease

Answers :			
1. A	2. A (mcm USA)	3. C	4. D
5. C	6. D	7. C	8. A

AIPG 2000

1. An autoimmune disease is all *except:*

A. Pemphigus vulgaris
B. Psoriasis
C. Lichen planus
D. Acne vulgaris

2. Palpable purpura is seen in all the following conditions *except*:

A. Giant cell arteritis
B. Cryoglobulinuria
C. Henoch-Schönlein purpura
D. Drug induced vasculitis

3. Regarding lichen planus all are true, *except*:

A. Hypopigmentation in residual disease
B. Lymphatic infiltration in supradermal layer
C. Ithcy polygonal, purple papule
D. Skin, hair and oral mucosa commonly involved

4. Regarding erythema multiforme, all are true *except*:

A. No vesicles
B. Target lesions are seen
C. Involves face and neck regions
D. Is a sign of internal malignancy

5. All of the following are seen in tuberous sclerosis, *except*:

A. Iris nodule
B. Renal cortical cyst
C. Rhabdomyoma of heart and lung
D. Adenoma sebaceum

6. All are true regarding psoriasis, *except*:

A. Head, neck and face are not involved
B. Arthritis is seen in 5% of cases
C. Abscess are seen in lesions
D. Non-scaly, red lesions are seen in infra mammary and natal regions

7. A patient has bullous eruption on lower limb and trunk. Biopsy shows sub epidermal bullae. The correct statement is:

A. Pemphigoid
B. Pehphigus vulgaris
C. Impetigo
D. Rule out internal malignancy

8. Which of the following is wrong statement?

A. Koilonychia in Vit B_{12} deficiency
B. Onycholysis in psoriasis
C. Mees lines in arsenic poisoning
D. Pterygium of nails in lichen planus

9. Which of the following is contraindicated in androgenic alopecia?

A. Testosterone
B. Cyproterone
C. Finasteride
D. Minoxidil

Answers :			
1. D	2. A	3. A	4. A
5. A	6. A	7. A	8. A
9. A			

AIPG 1999

1. Most common cause of air borne dermatitis in India is:

A. Parthenium
B. Crysophillous
C. Calotropis
D. Rothrangal

2. Patch test is read after:

A. 2 hours
B. 2 days
C. 2 weeks
D. 4 weeks

3. **Atopic dermatitis is diagnosed by:**
   A. Patch test B. Clinical examination
   C. Wood's lamp D. Increase IgE

4. **Cutaneous tuberculous secondary to underlying tissue is called as:**
   A. Scrofuloderma
   B. Lupus vulgaris
   C. Tuberculous verrucosa cutis
   D. Spina-ventosa

5. **Satellite lesions are seen in the following type of leprosy:**
   A. Tuberculoid leprosy
   B. Lepromatous leprosy
   C. Borderline tuberculoid leprosy
   D. Histoid leprosy

6. **Thalidomide is the drug of choice for:**
   A. Lepra type I reaction
   B. Lepra type II reaction
   C. Nerve abscess
   D. Nerve excision

7. **Permethrin is used in the treatment of:**
   A. Scabies B. Leprosy
   C. Body louse D. Leishmaniasis

8. **Chancroid may be caused by:**
   A. T. pallidium
   B. G. donovari
   C. Chlamydia trachomatis
   D. Herpes virus-hominis

9. **Cicatrical alopecia is seen in:**
   A. Tenia capitis
   B. Psoriasis
   C. Discoid lupus erythematosus
   D. Alopecia areata

Answers :

1. A	2. B	3. B	4. A
5. C	6. B	7. A	8. D
9. C			

AIPG 1998

1. **Target lesion in iris seen is:**
   A. Urticaria
   B. Erythema mutiformae
   C. Scabies
   D. Lichen planus

2. **A child with hypopigmented patch on cheek and no sensory loss and no scale, diagnosis is:**
   A. Indeterminate leprosy B. Scabies
   C. Pityriasis alba D. Alopecia areata

3. **Itchy polygonal violaceous papules seen in:**
   A. Psoriasis B. Pemphigus
   C. Lichen planus D. Pityriasis rosea

4. **Least common site involvement in psoriasis is:**
   A. Scalp B. Nail involvement
   C. CNS involvement D. Arthritis

5. **Gonococcus does not involve:**
   A. Testis B. Fallopian tube
   C. Epididymis D. Cervix

6. **True about syphilis is all *except*:**
   A. VDRL is sensitive but not specific
   B. Infection leads to life long immunity
   C. IgM and IgA
   D. T. pallidium when inoculated in rabbit produce progressive disease

Answers :

1. B	2. A	3. C	4. C
5. A	6. D		

AIPG 1997

1. **Staphylococcal infection causes all disease *except:***
   A. Impetigo
   B. Erysipelas
   C. Ecthyma
   D. Scaldy skin syndrome

2. **Donovanosis is caused by:**
   A. Calymatobacter granulomatis
   B. T. pertenue
   C. Chlamydia trachomatis
   D. H. ducreyi

3. **Skin biopsy in leprosy is characterized by:**
   A. Pariappendageal bacilli
   B. Pariappendageal lymphocytosis
   C. Perivascular lymphocytosis
   D. All of the above

4. Skin smear is negative in which leprosy?

A. Indeterminate
B. Neuritic
C. Lepromatous
D. Borderline

5. All lesions are seen in leprosy *except*:

A. Erythematous macule
B. Hypopigmented patch
C. Vesicles
D. Flat and raised patches

6. A 25 years old female has palatal ulcer and skin blister most likely diagnosis is:

A. Pemphigus vulgaris
B. Pemphigus follaceous
C. Dermatitis herpetiformis
D. Pemphigoid

Answers :

1. B	2. A	3. D	4. B
5. C	6. A		

AIPG 1996

1. Pseudo bubo is seen in:

A. Donovanosis
B. LGV
C. Chancroid
D. Syphilis

2. Frie test is done in:

A. Donovanosis
B. LGV
C. Syphilis
D. Leprosy

3. Discharging sinus is seen in:

A. Syphilis
B. Herpes
C. Actinomycosis
D. Molluscum contagiosum

4. WHO regime for paucibacillary leprosy:

A. 100 mg dapsone daily + rifampein monthly (600 mg)
B. Dapsone daily + rifampein daily
C. Dapsone + rifampein + clofazimine daily
D. Rifampein + clofazimine daily

5. Skin pigmentation and icthyosis like side effects are seen in:

A. Rifampecin
B. Clofazimine
C. Dapsone
D. Steroid

6. A patient has bullous lesion on Tzanck smear:

A. Langerhan's cells are seen
B. Acantholysis
C. Leucocytosis
D. Absence of melanin pigmented

7. Gonococcus resistant structure is:

A. Urethra
B. Testis
C. Fallopian tube
D. Ampulla

8. Underlying internal malignancy is not shown by:

A. Acanthosis nigricans and annular erythema
B. Bullous pyoderma and migratory necrotizing erythema
C. Granuloma annulare
D. Erythema gyratum repens

Answers :

1. A	2. B	3. C	4. A
5. B	6. B	7. B	8. C

AIPG 1995

1. DOC in type I lepra reaction with severe neuritis:

A. Thalidomide
B. Clofazimine
C. Dapsone
D. Systemic corticosteroid

2. Tinea unguium effects:

A. Nail fold
B. Nail plate
C. Joints
D. Inter digital space

3. Fordyce spots are:

A. Ectopic sebaceous gland
B. Ectopic eccrine glands
C. Ectopic apocrine glands
D. Ectopic mucosal glands

4. Flaky paint appearance of skin is seen in:

A. Dermatitis
B. Pellagra
C. Marasmus
D. Kwashiorkar

5. Acantholysis is seen in:

A. Epidermis
B. Epidermodermal junction
C. Dermis
D. In all the layers of skin

6. Lymphadenopathy is seen is all *except*:

A. Syphilis 1st stage
B. Donovanosis
C. LGV
D. Chancroid

Answers :

1. D	2. B	3. A	4. D
5. A	6. B		

AIPG 1994

1. **Primary bullous lesions is seen in which type of syphilis?**
   A. Primary B. Secondary
   C. Tertiary D. Congenital

2. **Bubos with multiple sinuses discharging into inguinal lymph nodes are seen in:**
   A. Chancroid B. Granuloma inguinale
   C. LGV D. Syphilis

3. **Treatment of choice in nodulocystic acne is:**
   A. Systemic steroids B. Retinoic acid
   C. Benzoyl peroxide D. Estrogen

4. **Treatment of choice in pustuar psoriasis in pregnancy:**
   A. Psoralin + UV therapy B. Systemic steroid
   C. Methotrexate D. Estrogen

5. **Multi drug therapy is given for:**
   A. Syphilis B. Leprosy
   C. Herpetiformis D. Ichthyosis vulgaris

6. **Drug induced pemphigus is seen in all *except*:**
   A. Penicillin B. Phenopthelein
   C. Iodine D. Furosemide

7. **Mouth lesions are seen in:**
   A. Psoriasis B. Lichen planus
   C. Basal cell C_A D. Ichthyosis vulgaris

Answers :

1. D	2. C	3. B	4. C
5. B	6. D	7. B	

AIPG 1993

1. **DOC for tenia unguium:**
   A. Amphotericin B B. Miconazole
   C. Griseofulvin D. Nystatin

2. **Test not used for diagnosis of syphilis:**
   A. VDRL B. TPI
   C. Reagin test D. Frei test

3. **Most common precipitant of contact dermatitis is:**
   A. Gold B. Nickel
   C. Silver D. Iron

4. **Toxic shock syndrome is caused by:**
   A. Staphylococcal infection B. Streptococcus
   C. Pseudomonas D. E. coli

5. **Inheritence of ichthyosis vulgaris is:**
   A. X-linked dominant
   B. X-linked recessive
   C. Autosomal dominant
   D. Autosomal recessive

6. **Single lesion in skin in seen in which type of leprosy?**
   A. Indeterminate leprosy B. BT
   C. BL D. LL

7. **Sabre tibia is seen in:**
   A. Scurvy B. Rickets
   C. Leprosy D. Syphilis

8. **Hyperpigmentation is not seen in:**
   A. Addison's disease **B.** Cushing's disease
   C. Grave's disease **D.** Hypothyroidism

Answers :

1. C	2. D	3. B	4. A
5. C	6. A	7. D	8. C

AIPG 1992

1. **Not transmitted sexually:**
   A. Syphilis B. T. pertenue
   C. Candida D. Gonorrhea

2. **Diagnostic method of choice in contact dermatitis:**
   A. Clinical examination B. Skin biopsy
   C. Tzanck smear D. Patch test

3. **Incorrect statement is: (Repeat in AIPG 2008)**
   A. VDRL titre decreases with treatment
   B. VDRL becomes positive after 21 days of infection
   C. FTA-ABS is earliest and most sensitive test
   D. Yaws and Pinta can be differentiated by serological tests

4. **DOC in primary syphilis is:**
   A. Corticosteroid
   B. Oral penicillin
   C. Benzathine penicillin
   D. Crystalline penicillin

5. **Kobner's phenomenon is seen in:**
   A. Pemphigus
   B. Darier's disease
   C. Lichen planus
   D. Tenia

6. **Tinea versicolor is caused by:**
   A. E. flaccosum
   B. Malassezia furfur
   C. T. rubrum
   D. T. schonlein

7. **Photochemotherapy is used in:**
   A. Pityriasis rosea
   B. Erythroderma
   C. Scabies
   D. Psoriasis

Answers :			
1. B	2. D	3. D	4. C
5. C	6. B	7. D	

AIPG 1991

1. **Kobner's phenomenon is seen in:**
   A. Lupus erythematous   B. Syphilis
   C. Lupus vulgaris   D. Psoriasis

2. **DOC for dermatitis herpetiformis is:**
   A. Steroids   B. Dapsone
   C. PUVA   D. Antihistaminic

3. **Intra epithelial bulla is seen in:**
   A. Pemphigus
   B. Pemphigoid
   C. Dermatitis herpetiformis
   D. Light eruption

4. **Herald patch is seen in:**
   A. Pityriasis rosea   B. P. alba
   C. Scarlet fever   D. Psoriasis

5. **Chloroquin is indicated in treatment of:** **(Repeat DPG 2009)**
   A. Pemphigus   B. Pemphigoid
   C. Psoriasis   D. DLE

6. **Not true of secondary syphilis:**
   A. May be asymptomatic
   B. Usually involve palms and soles
   C. Lymphadenopathy
   D. Vesicular lesions

7. **Lupus like picture is caused by all *except*:**
   A. Chloroquine   B. Procainamide
   C. Hydralazine   D. Isoniazid

Answers :			
1. D	2. B	3. A	4. A
5. D	6. D	7. A	

AIIMS

1990-2009

AIIMS MAY 2009

1. **Teatment of choice in Kawasaki disease:**
   A. IVIg   B. Aspirin
   C. Antibiotics   D. Oxygen

2. **Child with rash, palpable purpura, abdominal pain:**
   A. HSP   B. ITP
   C. Aplastic anemia   D. Septicaemia

3. **Patch test is based on what type of reaction?**
   A. Type 4 hypersensitivity reaction
   B. Type 1 hypersensitivity reaction
   C. Type 3 hypersensitivity reaction
   D. Type 2 hypersensitivity reaction

4. **Deposition of IgG in intercellular region of epidermis:**
   A. Dermatitis herptiformis
   B. Pemphigus vulgaris
   C. Bullous pemphigoid
   D. Lichen planus

5. **Granular subepidermal deposition of IgA:**
   A. Dermatitis herpetiformis
   B. Pemphigus vulgaris
   C. Bullous pemphigoid
   D. Linear IgA disease

6. **Neurofibromatosis all are true *except:***
   A. Autosomal recessive
   B. Scoliosis
   C. Neurofibroma
   D. Pheochromocytomas association

7. **Treponema pallidum isolated from CSF in:**
   A. Primary syphilis
   B. Secondary syphilis
   C. Tertiary syphilis
   D. Tabes dorsalis

Answers :

1. A	2. A	3. A	4. B
5. A	6. A	7. C	

AIIMS JANUARY 2009

1. **Lepromin test is:**
   A. Diagnostic
   B. Prognostic
   C. Treatment
   D. Epidemiologic evaluation

2. **Most common cause of mononeuritis multiplex in India:**
   A. TB B. RA
   C. Hansens D. Arsenic

3. **Glomus tumor found in:**
   A. Finger B. Liver
   C. Adrenal D. Pituitary

4. **A 9 years old female child, difficulty in climbing stairs since one month, gowers sign positive, rash on metacarpophalangeal joint investigation to be done:**
   A. ESR
   B. Rheu factor
   C. Raised creatinine kinase
   D. Electromyography

5. **Thalidomide used in all *except:***
   A. ENL
   B. HIV related neuropathy
   C. Multiple myeloma
   D. HIV related oral ulcers

6. **Cause of Reiter syndrome in India:**
   A. Urea plasma
   B. Histoplasma
   C. E. coli
   D. Shigella

7. **Not found in Reiter syndrome:**
   A. Oral ulcer
   B. Genital involvement
   C. E nodosum
   D. Skin rash

8. **A middle aged female presents with hypopigmented patch on the central part of the forehead. The chemical responsible is:**
   A. Hydroquinone
   B. Mono benzyl ether of hydroquinone
   C. Para tertiary butyl phenol
   D. Para tertiary butyl catechol

9. **A 2-month-old female child was brought with linear verrucous lesions on the trunk. Histopathology showed vacuolation of keratinocytes in the stratum spinosum and granulosum with IgG deposition. What is the most probable diagnosis?**
   A. Linear Darier's disease
   B. Incontinentia pigmenti
   C. Epidermolytic hyperkeratosis
   D. Ilven

Answers :

1. B	2. C	3. A	4. D
5. B	6. D	7. C	8. C
9. D			

AIIMS 2008

1. **Auspitz sign seen in:**
   A. Pustular psoriasis
   B. Plaque type psoriasis
   C. Lichen planus
   D. Pityriasis rubra pilaris

2. **Keratoderma blenorrhagicum is seen in:**
   A. Psoriasis
   B. Reiter's syndrome
   C. Syphilis
   D. Disseminated gonococcal infection

3. **Most common cause of plant induced dermatitis in India:**
   A. Poison ivy B. Parthenium
   C. Ragweed D. Cotton fibres

Answers :

1. B	2. B	3. B

AIIMS NOVEMBER 2007

1. **A child presents with non-blanching rash over the extensor aspect of arm with swelling over knee urine analysis show proteinuria 1 + and RBC 3 + on kidney biopsy which finding will be seen?**
   A. Fusion of podocytes
   B. ATN
   C. Depositions of IgA
   D. Thickening of membrane

2. **Most common brain tumor in NF1:**
   A. Optic glioma astrocytosis
   B. Glioblastoma multiforme
   C. Brain stem glioma
   D. Pilocytic astrocytoma

3. **Marker for Langerhan's cell histiocytosis:**
   A. CD-1a B. Cd-57
   C. Cd-34 D. Cd-54

4. **Vector of kala azar is:**
   A. Sand fly B. House bug
   C. Reduvid bug D. Tick

5. **A male patient C urethral discharge. On microscopy –only pus cells, no organism, leukocyte esterase (+) ve no glucose, no protein in urine. 50 wbc/HPF is seen. What is the likely diagnosis?**
   A. Chlamydia trachomatis
   B. Gonococcus
   C. Urea plasma urealyticum
   D. H.P.V.

6. **Scarring alopecia–caused by all *except*:**
   A. Lichen planus
   B. Pseudopelade
   C. DLE
   D. Alopecia areata

7. **Typhoid present with hair fall diagnosis is:**
   A. Telogen effuvium
   B. Anagen effluvium
   C. Alopecia areata
   D. Pseudopelade

Answers :

1. C	2. A	3. A	4. A
5. A	6. D	7. A	

AIIMS 2006

1. **Pityriasis rosea true is:**
   A. Self-limiting
   B. Chronic relapsing
   C. Life threatening infection
   D. Caused by dermatophytes

2. **A 3 years old child has eczematous dermatitis on extensor surfaces. His mother has a history of bronchial asthma. Diagnosis is:**
   A. Atopic dermatitis
   B. Contact dermatitis
   C. Seborrheic dermatitis
   D. Infantile eczematous dermatitis

3. **Chancre redux is a clinical feature of:**
   A. Early relapsing syphilis
   B. Late syphilis
   C. Chancroid
   D. Recurrent herpes simplex infection

4. **Anagen phase of hair indicates:**
   A. Phase of activity and growth
   B. Phase of transition
   C. Phase of resting
   D. Phase of degeneration

5. **Max Joseph space is histological feature of:**
   A. Psoriasis vulgaris B. Lichen planus
   C. Pityriasis rosea D. Parapsoriasis

6. **Ivermectin is indicated in treatment of:**
   A. Syphilis B. Scabies
   C. TB D. Dermatophytosis

7. **Following drug is not used in treatment of type 2 lepra reaction:**
   A. Chloroquine B. Thalidomide
   C. Cyclosporine D. Corticosteroids

8. **Main cytokine involved in ENL reaction:**
   A. IL2 B. Interferon gamma
   C. TNF alpha D. Macrophage colony stimulating factor

9. Following test is not used for diagnosis of leprosy:

A. Lepromin test B. Slit skin smear
C. FNAC D. Skin biopsy

10. Air borne contact dermatitis can be diagnosed by:

A. Skin biopsy
B. Patch test
C. Prick test
D. Estimation of serum IGE levels

Answers :

1. A	2. A	3. A	4. A
5. B	6. B	7. C	8. C
9. C	10. B		

AIIMS 2005

1. Exclamation hair mark is feature of:

A. Telogen effluvium
B. Androgenetic alopecia
C. Alopecia areata
D. Alopecia mucinosa

2. Paurriers microabscesses is a histo feature of:

A. Sarcoidosis
B. TB
C. Mycosis fungoides
D. Pityriasis lichenoides chronica

3. Adenoma sebaceum is a feature of:

A. Neurofibromatosis
B. Tuberous sclerosis
C. Xanthomatosis
D. Incontinentia pigmenti

4. A 27 years old male had burning micturition and urethral discharge. After 4 weeks he developed joint pains involving both knees and ankles, redness of eye and skin lesion. The most probable diagnosis is:

A. Psoriasis vulgaris
B. Reiter's syndrone
C. Behcet's syndrome
D. Sarcoidosis

5. Which one of the following is treatment of choice of dermatitis herpetiformis?

A. Corticosteroids B. Dapsone
C. Methotrexate D. Retinoids

6. A 6 months old infant presented with multiple papule and exudative lesions on face, scalp, trunk and few vesicles on palms and soles for 2 weeks. His mother had history of itchy lesions. The most likely diagnosis is:

A. Scabies
B. Infantile eczema
C. Infantile seborrheic dermatitis
D. Impetigo contagiosa

7. Punch purpura is diagnostic of:

A. Systemic primary amyloidosis
B. Secondary systemic amyloidosis
C. Idiopathic thrombocytopenic purpura
D. Drug induced purpura

Answers :

1. C	2. C	3. B	4. B
5. B	6. A	7. A	

AIIMS NOVEMBER 2003

1. A 30 years old male patient has a large, spreading and exuberant ulcer with bright red granulation tissue over the glans penis. There was no lymphadenopathy. The most likely causative organism is:

A. Treponema pallidum
B. Herpes simplex virus type 1
C. Herpes simplex virus type 2
D. Calymmatobacterium granulomatis

2. A 22 years old male patient presents with a complaint of severe itching and white scaly lesions in the groin for past month. Which of the following is most likely to be the causative agent?

A. Trichophyton rubrum B. Candida albicans
C. Candida glabrata D. Malassezia furfur

3. A 16 years old student reported for the evaluation of multiple hypopigmented macules on the trunk and limbs. All of the following tests are useful in making a diagnosis of leprosy, *except*:

A. Sensation testing
B. Lepromin test
C. Slit smears
D. Skin biopsy

4. A 12 years old boy had a gradually progressive plaque on a buttock for the last 3 years. The plaque was 15 cm in diameter, annular in shape, with crusting and induration at the periphery and

scarring at the center. The most likely diagnosis:

A. Tinea corporis
B. Granuloma annulare
C. Lupus vulgaris
D. Borderline leprosy

5. A 24 years old man had multiple, small hypopigmented macules on the upper chest and back for the last three months. The macules were circular, arranged around follicles and many had coalesced to form large sheets. The surface of the macules showed fine scaling. He had similar lesions one year ago which subsided with treatment. The most appropriate investigation to confirm the diagnosis is:

A. Potassium hydroxide preparation of scales
B. Slit skin smear from discrete macules
C. Tzanck test
D. Skin biopsy of coalesced macules

6. A 22 years old woman developed small itchy wheals after physical exertion, walking in the sun, eating hot spicy food and when she was angry. The most likely diagnosis is:

A. Chronic idiopathic utricaria
B. Heat urticaria
C. Solar urticaria
D. Cholinergic urticaria

7. A 45 years old male had multiple hypoaesthetic mildly erythematous large plaques with elevated margins on trunk and extremities. His ulnar and lateral popliteal nerves on both sides were enlarged. The most probable diagnosis is:

A. Lepromatous leprosy
B. Borderline leprosy
C. Borderline tuberculoid leprosy
D. Borderline lepromatous leprosy

Answers :

1. D	2. A	3. B	4. C
5. A	6. D	7. C	

AIIMS MAY 2003

1. The following drug is indicated in the treatment of pityriasis versicolor:

A. Ketoconazole
B. Metronidazole
C. Griseofulvin
D. Chloroquine

2. A 24 years old male presents to an STD clinic with a single painless ulcer on external genitalia. The choice of laboratory test to look for the etiological agent would be:

A. Scrappings from ulcer for culture on chocolate agar with antibiotic supplement
B. Serology for detection of specific IgM antibodies
C. Scrappings from ulcer for dark field microscopy
D. Scrappings from ulcer for tissue culture

3. Podophyllum resin is indicated in the treatment of:

A. Psoriasis
B. Pemphigus
C. Condyloma acuminata
D. Condylomata lata

4. A 24 years old female has flaccid bullae in the skin and oral erosions. Histopathology shows intra-epidermal acantholytic blister. The most likely diagnosis is:

A. Pemphigoid
B. Erythema multiforme
C. Pemphigus vulgaris
D. Dermatitis herpetiformis

Answers :

1. A	2. C	3. C	4. C

AIIMS NOVEMBER 2002

1. A 45 years old male has multiple grouped vesicular lesions present on the T10 segment dermatome associated with pain. The most likely diagnosis is:

A. Herpes zoster
B. Dermatitis herpetiformis
C. Herpes simplex
D. Scabies

2. A 28 years old patient has multiple grouped papulovesicular lesions on both elbows, knees, buttocks and upper back associated with severe itching. The most likely diagnosis is:

A. Pemphigus vulgaris
B. Bullous pemphigoid
C. Dermatitis herpetiformis
D. Herpes zoster

3. A child has multiple itchy papular lesions on the genitalia and fingers. Similar lesions are also seen

in younger brother. Which of the following is most possible diagnosis?

A. Papular urticaria
B. Scabies
C. Atopic dermatitis
D. Allergic contact dermatitis

4. Which layer of epidermis is underdeveloped in the VLBW infants in the initial 7 days?

A. Stratum germinativum
B. Stratum granulosum
C. Stratum lucidum
D. Stratum corneum

5. Scabies, an infection of the skin caused by sarcoptes scabie, is an example of:

A. Water borne disease
B. Water washed disease
C. Water based disease
D. Water related disease

Answers :

1. A	2. C	3. B	4. D	5. B

AIIMS MAY 2002

1. Treatment of pustular psoriasis is:

A. Thalidomide B. Retinoids
C. Hydroxyurea D. Methotrexate

2. A patient presents with erythematous scaly lesions on extensor aspect of elbows and knee. The clinical diagnosis is got by:

A. Auspitz sign B. KOH smear
C. Tzanck smear D. Skin biopsy

3. Actinic keratosis is seen in:

A. Basal cell carcinoma
B. Squamous cell carcinoma
C. Malignant melanoma
D. Epithelial cell carcinoma

4. A 30 years old female presents with history of itching under right breast. On examination annular ring lesion was present under the breast. The diagnosis is:

A. Trichophyton rubrum B. Candida albicans
C. Epidermophyton D. Microsporum

5. Wood's lamp light is used in the diagnosis of:

A. Tinea capitis B. Candida albicans
C. Histoplasma D. Cryptococcus

6. A patient presented with multiple nodulocystic lesions on the face. The drug of choice is:

A. Retinoids B. Antibiotics
C. Steroids D. UV light

Answers :

1. B	2. A	3. B	4. A
5. A	6. A		

AIIMS NOVEMBER 2001

1. Acne vulgaris is due to involvement of:

A. Sebaceous gland
B. Pilosebaceous gland
C. Eccrine gland
D. Apocrine gland

2. A patient with psoriasis was started on systemic steroids. After stopping treatment patient developed generalied pustules all over his body, the most likely cause is:

A. Drug induced reactions
B. Pustular psoriasis
C. Bacterial infection
D. Septicemia

3. A patient presents with scarring alopecia, thinned nails, hypopigmented macular lesions over trunk and oral mucosa. The diagnosis is:

A. Psoriasis B. Leprosy
C. Lichen planus D. Pemphigus

4. A young boy presented with lesion over his right buttock which had peripheral scaling and central scarring. The investigation of choice would be:

A. Tzanck smear B. KOH preparation
C. Biopsy D. Saboraud's agar

Answers :

1. B	2. B	3. C	4. C

AIIMS MAY 2001

1. An 8 years old boy presents with a well defined annular lesion over the buttock with central scarring that is gradually progressing over the last 8 months. The diagnosis is:

A. Annular psoriasis

B. Lupus vulgaris
C. Tinea corporis
D. Chronic granulomatous disease

2. The characteristic nail finding in lichen planus is:

A. Pitting
B. Pterygium
C. Beau's lines
D. Hyperpigmentation of the nails

3. An adult presents with oval scaly hypopigmented macule over the chest and the back. The diagnosis is:

A. Leprosy
B. Lupus vulgaris
C. Pityriasis versicolor
D. Lichen planus

4. A 40 years old farmer with a history of recurrent attacks of porphyria complains of itching when exposes to the sun and maculopapular rash on sun exposed areas, his symptoms are exaggerated in the summer. The diagnosis is:

A. Seborrheic dermatitis
B. Contact dermatitis
C. Psoriasis
D. Porphyria cutanea tarda

5. In an 8 days old child with no history of consanguinity in the parents, the mother reports blisters and bleeding off of the skin at the site of handling and pressure. There was a similar history in the previous child which proved to be fatal. The diagnosis is:

A. Bullous pemphigoid
B. Congenital syphilis
C. Congenital epidermolysis bullosa
D. Letterer-Siwe disease

Answers :

1. B **2. B** **3. C** **4. D** **5. C**

AIIMS NOVEMBER 2000

1. A child presents with a solitary white well defined patch on his right thigh. What is the diagnosis?

A. Piebaldism
B. Acral vitiligo
C. Nevus achromicus
D. Albinism

2. Babloo, a 4 years old boy, presents with history of seizures, on examination there is hypopigmented patches on his face. There is mental retardation also. What is most likely diagnosis?

A. Neurofibromatosis
B. Tuberous sclerosis
C. Sturge-Weber syndrome
D. Incontinentia pigmenti

3. A patient gets recurrent urticaria while doing exercise and on exposure to sunlight. Which of the following is the most likely cause?

A. Chronic idiopathic urticaria
B. Universal sermographism
C. Cholinergic urticaria
D. Photo dermatitis

4. Babloo, 5 years old, presents with small hypopigmented scaly macules on his cheek. *Some of his classmates also have similar lesion.* Which of the following is the most probable diagnosis? ‡‡

A. Pityriasis rosea
B. Pityriasis versicolor
C. Indeterminate leprosy
D. Pityriasis alba

(Note that the disease can spread: So obviously it's an infection.)

Answers :

1. C **2. B** **3. C** **4. B**

AIIMS JUNE 2000

1. Nikolsky sign is positive in all *except*:

A. Pemphigus
B. Bullous pemphigoid
C. Toxic epidermonecrolysis
D. Staphylococcal scalded skin syndrome

2. Most common cause of allergic contact dermatitis in Indian females is:

A. Vegetables
B. Nail polish remover
C. Nail polish
D. Detergents

3. Lepromin test is positive in:

A. Lepromatous leprosy
B. Indeterminate leprosy
C. Tuberculoid leprosy
D. Histoid leprosy

Answers :

1. B **2. D** **3. C**

AIIMS NOVEMBER 1999

1. **Satellite lesions are seen in:**
   A. Indeterminate leprosy
   B. Borderline tuberculoid leprosy
   C. Borderline leprosy
   D. Lepromatous leprosy

2. **A boy comes from Bihar with anaesthetic, hypopigmented, atrophic patch over face. The diagnosis is:**
   A. Borderline leprosy
   B. Pityriasis versicolor
   C. Pityriasis alba
   D. Indeterminate leprosy

3. **Lymphogranuloma venerum is caused by:**
   A. Chlamydia trachomatis
   B. Hemophillus ducrei
   C. Human T cell lymphoma virus type II
   D. Donovania granulomatis

4. **Condylomata lata is seen in:**
   A. Primary syphilis
   B. Secondary syphilis
   C. Congenital syphilis
   D. Tertiary syphilis

Answers :

1. B **2. D** **3. A** **4. B**

AIIMS JUNE 1999

1. **A 3 years old female child develops umbilicated nodules over face following a trivial viral infection the probable diagnosis is:**
   A. Lichen planus
   B. Chicken pox
   C. Scabies
   D. Molluscum contagiosum

2. **A 10 years old child has violaceous papule and pterygium of nails, the diagnosis is:**
   A. Psoriasis B. Lichen planus
   C. Pemphigus D. Pemphigoid

3. **A 23 years old lady develops brown macular lesions over bridge of nose and cheeks following exposure to light. The probable diagnosis is:**
   A. Chloasma
   B. Acne rosacea
   C. Systemic lupus erythematosis
   D. Photodermatitis

4. **A 10 years old child has hypopigmented, multiple scaly patch over face. The likely diagnosis is:**
   A. Pityriasis alba
   B. Tinea versicolor
   C. Leprosy
   D. Indeterminate leprosy

Answers :

1. D **2. B** **3. A** **4. A**

AIIMS DECEMBER 1998

1. **Tuberculossis of skin is called as:**
   A. Scrofuloderma B. Lupus pernio
   C. Lupus profundus D. Lupus vulgaris

2. **Kerion is seen in:**
   A. Pityriasis B. Dermatophytosis
   C. Candidiasis D. Trichomoniasis

3. **Comedones are seen in:**
   A. Pityriasis **B.** Lichen planus
   C. Adenoma sebaceum **D.** Acne vulgaris

4. **An 8 years old patient presenting with hypopigmented scaly lesion on the face. The diagnosis is:**
   A. Pityriasis alba
   B. Tuberculoid leprosy
   C. Vitiligo
   D. Indeterminate leprosy

5. **An eight years old boy presents with multiple umbilicated papules on trunk. Diagnosis is:**
   A. Molluscum contagiosum B. Chicken pox
   C. Herpes zoster D. Dermatophytosis

6. **An 8 years old boy presents with boggy swelling and easily pluckable hair, diagnosis is:**
   A. Tinea capitis B. Alopecia areata
   C. Tuberculoid leprosy D. Pityriasis alba

Answers :

1. D **2. B** **3. D** **4. A**
5. A **6. A**

AIIMS JUNE 1998

1. **All are features of secondary syphilis, *except*:**
   A. Papulosquamous lesion
   B. Bullous lesion
   C. Nodular lesion
   D. Lichenoid type lesion

2. **Type of nail changes in lichen planus is:**
   A. Pitting
   B. Pterygium
   C. Subungual hyperkeratosis
   D. Onycholysis

3. **A 6 years old child from Tamil Nadu presents with a solitary non-anaesthetic patch on face, the possible diagnosis is:**
   A. Pityriasis alba
   B. Indeterminate leprosy
   C. Pityriasis versicolor
   D. Tinea infection

4. **A child has umbilicated nodule on face, the diagnosis is:**
   A. Seborrheic dermatitis
   B. Chicken pox
   C. Tinea
   D. Molluscum contagiosum

Answers :

1. B 2. B 3. B 4. D

AIIMS DECEMBER 1997

1. **Acantholysis is due destruction of:**
   A. Epidermis
   B. Subepidermis
   C. Intercellular substance
   D. Basement membrane

2. **Most potent anti-leprotic drug is:**
   A. Clofazimine B. Dapsone
   C. Rifampicin D. Norfloxacin

3. **Anti leprotic drug used in lepra reaction is:**
   A. Acedapsone B. Rifampicin
   C. Dapsone D. Clofazimine

4. **Genital ulcer is seen in all, *except*:**
   A. Granuloma inguinale
   B. LGV
   C. Donovanosis
   D. Syphilis

5. **Annular herald's patch is seen in:**
   A. Psoriasis B. Pityriasis rosea
   C. Pityriasis alba D. Nocardiasis

Answers :

1. C 2. C 3. D 4. B 5. B

AIIMS JUNE 1997

1. **All are features of secondary syphilis, *except*:**
   A. Papule B. Papulosquamous
   C. Bullae D. Nodules

2. **Which layer of skin causes vesicular changes in case of burn:**
   A. Basal layer B. Papillary layer
   C. Epidermis D. Dermis

3. **"Target lesions" are characteristics of:**
   A. Dermatitis herpetiformis
   B. Sulpha drug reaction
   C. Lichen planus
   D. Erythema multiforme

4. **A 56 years old male having painful bullous lesion in lower extremity, the most likely diagnosis is:**
   A. Pemphigus vulgaris
   B. Bullous pemphigoid
   C. Necrotising pemphigus
   D. Contact eczema

5. **Drug of choice for dermatitis herpetiformis is:**
   A. Dapsone B. Griseofulvin
   C. Rifampicin D. Ketoconazole

6. **Nodular scabies is found in:**
   A. Web space of finger B. Axilla
   C. Scrotum D. Abdomen

Answers :

1. C 2. D 3. D 4. B
5. A 6. C

AIIMS FEBRUARY 1997

1. **Recurrent oral ulcers with pain erythematous halo around them, the diagnosis is:**
   A. Aphthous ulcer B. Herpes
   C. Chicken pox D. Measles

2. Which is not a manifestation of secondary syphilis?

A. Vesicle and bullae
B. Hyperpigmented macules
C. Nodules
D. Rashes

3. Skin tuberculosis which involves skin after involving lymph nodes:

A. Scrofuloderma
B. Lupus vulgaris
C. Lupus erythematosus
D. Lupus pernio

Answers :

1. A 2. A 3. A

AIIMS SEPTEMBER 1996

1. Best method of treatment of ulnar nerve abscess in a case of leprosy is:

A. Incision and drainage
B. High dose of steroid
C. Thalidomide

2. A 20 years old male develops multiple ulcer over prepuce and glans, which are painful along with suppurative inguinal lymphadenopathy, 5 days after having sexual intercourse with a lady, most probable diagnosis is:

A. Molluscum contagiosum
B. Anaerobic streptococci
C. Herpes
D. Chancroid

3. A boggy swelling over scalp with easily pluckable hairs in a child, the investigation done is:

A. Giemsa staining
B. Bacterial culture
C. KOH preparation

4. A 7 years old child with recurrent scaly, hypopigmented patch on the face, diagnosis is:

A. Early vitiligo
B. Indeterminate leprosy
C. Pityriasis alba
D. Pityriasis rosea

Answers :

1. B 2. D 3. C 4. C

AIIMS DECEMBER 1995

1. Intra epidermal bulla is seen in:

A. Pemphigoid
B. Pemphigus
C. Dermatitis herpetiformis
D. Light reaction

2. Photochemotherapy is useful in:

A. Tinea captitis B. Psoriasis
C. Lichen planus D. Icthyosis vulgaris

3. Pseudo bubo are seen in:

A. Donovanosis B. Chancroid
C. LGV D. Syphilis

4. Papulovesicular lesions on face, trunk palm and sole in a 9 months old child is seen in:

A. Seborrheic dermatitis B. Atopic dermatitis
C. Scabies D. Drug reaction

5. Gold poisoning leading to exfoliative dermatitis is treated with:

A. Chloroquine B. Steroid
C. Antibiotics D. Antihistaminics

Answers :

1.B 2. B 3. A 4. C 5. B

AIIMS MAY 1995

1. Treatment of choice of nodulocystic acne is:

A. Erythromycin B. Isoretinoin
C. Tetracycline D. PUVA

Answer :

1. B

AIIMS DECEMBER 1994

1. What does not cause tinea capitis?

A. Epidermophyton floccosum
B. Microsporum
C. Trichophyton violaceum
D. Trichophyton rubrum

2. Most common nerve involved in leprosy is:

A. Ulnar
B. Median
C. Radial
D. Sciatic

3. **A 19-year-old girl has multiple papulopustular erythematous lesion on face and neck. The likely diagnosis is:**
   A. Acne rosacea B. Acne vulgaris
   C. Pityriasis versicolor D. Lupus vulgaris

4. **Most common cause of air borne contact dermatitis in India is:**
   A. Parthenium B. Garden grass
   C. Oleander D. Yellow oleander

5. **A patient presents with single hypopigmented anaesthetic patch with satellite lesion on forearm. The most likely diagnosis is:**
   A. Indeterminate leprosy
   B. Tuberculoid leprosy
   C. Neuritic leprosy
   D. Lepramatous leprosy

Answers :

1. A 2. A 3. B 4. A 5. B

AIIMS MAY 1994

1. **Boggy swelling with hair easily pluckable in a 10 years old child, investigation of choice is:**
   A. Biopsy B. X-ray skull
   C. KOH smear D. Tzank smear

2. **Treatment of nodulocystic acne is:**
   A. Erythromycin B. Isotretinoin
   C. Tetracycline D. Corticosteroid

3. **Treatment of lepra-I reaction:**
   A. Thalidomide
   B. Corticosteroids
   C. Increase in dapsone dose
   D. Clofazimine

Answers :

1. C 2. B 3. B

AIIMS NOVEMBER 1993

1. **Multiple, painful ulcers over glans penis without induration is suggestive of:**
   A. LGV
   B. Granuloma inguinale
   C. Chancroid
   D. Secondary syphilis

2. **Treatment of choice of pediculosis corporis is:**
   A. 3 applications of benzene hexachloride
   B. One application of benzyl benzoate
   C. 4 applications of benzyl benzoate
   D. Disinfection of clothes only

3. **An 8 years old child has localized, non-cicatrical alopecia over scalp with itching and scales. The diagnosis is:**
   A. Tinea barbae B. Alopecia areata
   C. Tinea capitis D. Lichen planus

4. **Average duration of treatment in multibacillary leprosy is:**
   A. 1 year B. 2 years
   C. 3 years D. Life long

5. **Cell mediated immunity is maximally suppressed in:**
   A. Borderline leprosy
   B. Lepromatous leprosy
   C. Tuberculoid leprosy
   D. Indeterminate type

Answers :

1. C 2. D 3. C 4. A 5. B

AIIMS MAY 1993

1. **In generalized lichen planus, treatment of choice is:**
   A. Topical salicyclic acid
   B. Ultraviolet rays
   C. Systemic steroids
   D. Erythromycin

2. **E.N.L. is seen in which type of leprosy:**
   A. BT B. LL
   C. TT D. Indeterminate

3. **Lepromin test is strongly positive in:**
   A. BT B. TT
   C. BL D. LL

4. **About dermatophytes, all are true, *except*:**
   A. Candida albicans usually causes systemic infections
   B. Superficial layer of skin involved
   C. Microsporum does not involve nail
   D. Epidermophyton does not involve hair

Answers :

1. C **2. B** **3. B** **4. A**

AIIMS DECEMBER 1992

1. **Recalcitrant pustular acne is treated by:**
   A. Steroids B. Retinoids
   C. Oral erythromycin D. Oral tetracycline

2. **Treatment of choice of dermatitis herpetiformis is:**
   A. Chloroquine B. Acyclovir
   C. Dapsone (DDS) D. Steroids

3. **Tinea capitis is caused by all, *except*:**
   A. Epidermophyton floccosum
   B. Microsporum canis
   C. Trichophyton schoenleinii
   D. Trichophyton rubrum

4. **Drug of choice in erythema nodosum leprosum:**
   A. Steroid B. Thalidomide
   C. Clofazimine D. Aspirin

5. **Erythema nodosum is seen in all, *except*:**
   A. Rheumatoid arthritis B. Tuberculosis
   C. Enteric fever D. Aspirin therapy

6. **Nails are not involved in:**
   A. Psoriasis
   B. Tinea
   C. Lichen planus
   D. Discoid lupus erythematosus (DLE)

Answers :

1. B **2. C** **3. A** **4. B**
5. D **6. D**

AIIMS JUNE 1992

1. **Ringworm fungi live in:**
   A. Stratum corneum
   B. Skin surface lipid film
   C. Dermis
   D. Prickle cell layer of epidermis

2. **Umbilicated, pearly white papules are seen in:**
   A. Plane warts
   B. Molluscum contagiosum
   C. Chickenpox
   D. Herpes genitalis

3. **Alopecia areata is presumed to be:**
   A. Androgenic in nature
   B. Autoimmune in etiology
   C. Part of the lichenoid spectrum
   D. Infective in nature

4. **Erythema nodosum leprosum is seen in:**
   A. Tuberculoid leprosy
   B. Borderline tuberculoid leprosy
   C. Lepromatous leprosy
   D. Indeterminate leprosy

Answers :

1. A **2. B** **3. B** **4. C**

AIIMS DECEMBER 1991

1. **Subepithelial bullae are seen in all *except*:**
   A. Dermatitis herpetiformis
   B. Pemphigoid
   C. Pemphigus
   D. Molluscum contagiosum

2. **Drug of choice of pustular psoriasis is:**
   A. PUVA B. Methotrexate
   C. Steroid D. Cyclophosphamide

3. **Disease commonly involving nails is:**
   A. Psoriasis B. SLE
   C. Pemphigus D. Rheumatoid arthritis

4. **Acantholysis is a feature of:**
   A. Dermatitis herpetiformis B. Viral warts
   C. Pemphigoid D. Pemphigus

5. **Herald patch is seen in:**
   A. Lichen planus B. Pityriasis rosea
   C. Pityriasis alba D. Pemphigus

Answers :

1. C **2. B** **3. A** **4. D** **5. B**

AIIMS JUNE 1991

1. **Most common age group to suffer from infection by tinea cruris is:**
   A. Adult male B. Adult female
   C. Male child D. Infant

2. **Acantholysis is seen in:**
   A. Pemphigoid
   B. Pemphigus vulgaris
   C. Erythema multiforme
   D. Dermatitis herpetiformis

3. **Podophyllin is treated of choice in:**
   A. Condyloma lata
   B. Plain warts
   C. Plantar warts
   D. Condyloma acuminata

4. **Erythema nodosum is not seen:**
   A. Sulfonamide therapy
   B. Primary TB
   C. Giant cell arteritis
   D. Streptococcal infection

5. **Mycosis fungoides is best treated by:**
   A. Electron beam therapy
   B. 5-FU cream
   C. Surgery
   D. Intravenous doxorubein (Adriamycin)

6. **Normal turnover time for epidermis is:‡**
   A. 2 weeks B. 4 weeks
   C. 6 weeks D. 8 weeks

7. **Lepromatous leprosy is characterized by all, *except*:**
   A. Gynaecomastia
   B. Saddle nose
   C. Loss of eyebrows
   D. Perforating ulcer

Answers :

1. A	2. B	3. D	4. A
5. A	6. D	7. D	

AIIMS 1990

1. **Mucous membrane lesions are seen in:**
   A. Pemphigus B. Pemphigoid
   C. Impetigo D. D. herpatiformis

2. **Herald patch is seen in:**
   A. Pityriasis versicolor B. P. alba
   C. P. rosea D. Psoriasis

3. **Griseofulvin is used in all *except*:**
   A. Tinea capitis
   B. Tinea versicolor and candida
   C. Tinea corporis
   D. Tinea unguium

4. **Streptomycin is useful in treatment of:**
   A. Granuloma venerum/Inguinale
   B. LGV
   C. Syphilis
   D. Chancroid

Answers :

1. A	2. C	3. B	4. A

PGI MCQs (2000-2009)

PGI 2009

1. **True regarding Munro micro abscesses:**
   A. Seen in stratum corneum
   B. Eosinophils only
   C. Debris consists of neutrophils+ eosinophils
   D. Associated pustule may be present
   E. Seen in psoriasis

2. **Subepidermal blister occurs in:**
   A. Bullous pemphigoid
   B. Pemphigus vulgaris
   C. Hailey-Hailey
   D. Darier's disease
   E. Acanthosis nigricans

3. **True about apocrine gland:**
   A. Found in axilla and groin
   B. Fordyce spots are seen
   C. Are odoriferous
   D. Modification of sebaceous gland

4. **Stratum lucidum is:**
   A. Layer sandwiched between stratum corneum and granulosum
   B. Between stratum germinativum and basale
   C. Seen all over body
   D. Seen on the palm and sole

5. **Normal commensals of skin:**
   A. Staph aureus
   B. Candida

C. Acinetobacter
D. P. acnes

Answers :

1. A, D, E 2. A 3. C 4. A
5. D

PGI 2008

1. **Pitted keratolysis is caused by:**
A. Corynebacterium B. Staph aureus
C. M leprae D. Sarcoidosis

2. **Circle of hebra is seen in:**
A. Scabies B. Pityriasis alba
C. Sarcoidosis D. Leprosy

Answers :

1. A 2. A

PGI 2007

1. **Which of the following is seen in psoriasis?**
A. Auspitz sign
B. Grenz zone
C. Munro abscess
D. Suprapapillary thinning

2. **Non-cicatricial alopecia is seen in:**
A. Psoriasis B. Lichen planus
C. Favus D. Alopecia areata

3. **Interferon therapy can be caused for:**
A. SCC B. BCC
C. Melanoma D. Bowen's disease

4. **Normal resident of human hair follicle:**
A. Propionobacterium B. Staphylococcus
C. Malassezia D. Candida

5. **Nail involvement is seen in:**
A. Psoriasis B. Lichen planus
C. Fungal infection D. Alopecia areata

Answers :

1. A,C,D 2. A,D 3. A,B,C 4. A,B,C
5. A,B,C,D

1. **Mucosa is involved in:**
A. Psoriasis B. Lichen planus
C. Alopecia D. Scabies
E. Porphyria

2. **Miliaria is a disorder of:**
A. Sebaceous gland B. Apocrine gland
C. Merocrine gland D. Holocrine gland
E. Eccrine gland

3. **Cicatricial alopecia is seen in:**
A. DLE B. Psoriasis
C. Alopecia areata D. Lichen planus
E. SLE

4. **Nail is involved in:**
A. Psoriasis B. Lichen planus
C. Fungal infection D. Alopecia (areata)
E. Viral infection

Answers :

1. B 2. E 3. A,D 4. A,B,C,D

PGI 2006

1. **Drugs used in MRSA:**
A. Quinopristine/Dalfopristine
B. Linezolid
C. Teicoplanin
D. Penicillin
E. Piperacillin

2. **Zn deficieincy causes:**
A. Cardiomyopathy B. Reduced growth
C. Gonadal atrophy D. Mental retardation

3. **N gonorrhoea causes:**
A. Urethritis B. Salpingitis
C. Cervicitis D. Vaginitis
E. Conjunctivitis

4. **ANCA is + in:**
A. Wegener's granulomatis
B. Churg-Strauss syndrome
C. Microscopic PAN
D. Goodpasture's syndrome

5. **Chancroid all are true *except:***
A. IP is 30 days B. Painful LN
C. Fever D. Ulcer
E. Balanitis

6. **A patient with glutein enteropathy can eat:**
   A. Rice
   B. Barley
   C. Oat
   D. Corn
   E. Rye

7. **HP finding in psoriasis:**
   A. Munro abscess
   B. Suprapapillary thinning
   C. Grenz zone
   D. Pautrier's abscess
   E. Hyperkeratosis

8. **Most common type of skin TB:**
   A. Lupus vulgaris
   B. Scrofuloderma
   C. TBVC
   D. E indurativum

9. **Wood's lamp is used for:**
   A. P versicolor
   B. Vitiligo
   C. Porphyria
   D. Psoriasis
   E. L planus

Answers :

1. A,B,C	2. B,C	3. A,B,C, E	4. A,B,C
5. A	6. A,C,D	7. A,B,E	8. A
9. A,B,C			

PGI 2005

1. **Treatment of acne:**
   A. 13 cis retinoic acid
   B. Minocycline
   C. Erythromycin
   D. Dapsone
   E. Rifampicin

2. **Which of the following are fungal infections of the skin?**
   A. Sporotrichosis
   B. Molluscum
   C. Madura foot
   D. Tinea
   E. Erysipelas

3. **Which of the following are bacterial infections of the skin?**
   A. Pyoderma gangrenosum
   B. Piedra
   C. Impetigo
   D. Impetigo herpetiformis
   E. Echthyma

4. **Causes of erythroderma:**
   A. P alba
   B. P versicolor
   C. Psoriasis
   D. Lichen planus
   E. Eczema

5. **Treatment of T unguium:**
   A. Fluconazole
   B. Itraconazole
   C. Terbinafine
   D. Neomycin

6. **Treatment of psoriasis:**
   A. PUVA
   B. Mtx
   C. Systemic steroids
   D. Femicycline
   E. Terbinafine

7. **ENL is seen in:**
   A. Indeterminate leprosy
   B. BT
   C. LL
   D. BL

8. **Kaposi varicelliform eruption is seen in:**
   A. AD
   B. Darier's
   C. Lichen planus
   D. Varicella

9. **P vulgaris like presentation is seen in:**
   A. Paraneoplastic pemphigus
   B. Bullous pemhigoid
   C. Dermatitis herpetiformis
   D. EB acquisita

10. **Hypopigmented patch is seen in:**
   A. N depigmentosus
   B. Freckles
   C. N of ito
   D. N of ota
   E. N anemicus

Answers:

1. A,B,C	2. A,C,D	3. A,C,E	4. C,D,E
5. A,B,C	6. A,B,C	7. C,D	8. A,B
9. A	10. A,E		

PGI 2004

1. **Intraepidermal vesicle is seen in:**
   A. P vulgaris
   B. Paraneoplastic pemphigus
   C. Dermatitis herpetiformis
   D. Congenital EB
   E. Trauma

2. **Hypo-depigmented macules are seen in:**
   A. N ito
   B. N depigmentosus
   C. N of ota
   D. N anemicus
   E. Freckles

3. **Skin manifestation of TB are:**
   A. Lupus vulgaris
   B. L pernio
   C. Scrofuloderma
   D. Butcher's warts

4. **ENL is seen in:**
A. BL
B. LL
C. BT
D. TT

5. **True about primary chancre is:**
A. Multiple
B. Painless solitary ulcer
C. Most infective stage
D. Heals automatically
E. Peniclillin is the drug of choice

6. **Adult scabies is characterized by involvement of:**
A. Palms and soles
B. Face
C. Anterior abdomen
D. Web space
E. Genitalia

7. **Koebner's phenomenon is seen in:**
A. Lichen planus
B. Warts
C. Behcet's syndrome
D. Psoriasis
E. Vitiligo

8. **True about lichen planus is:**
A. Basal cell degeneration
B. Colloid bodies are seen
C. Epidermal hyperplasia can be seen
D. Wickham stria are seen
E. Autoimmune

9. **Minor features of atopic dermatitis are:**
A. Dry skin
B. Pruritus
C. Morgan fold
D. P alba
E. Dermographism

10. **True about lupus vulgaris:**
A. Apple jelly nodules
B. TB of skin and mucus membrane
C. Also called scrofuloderma
D. ATT helpful

11. **Cicatricial alopecia is seen in:**
A. DLE
B. SLE
C. Syphilis
D. Psoriasis

Answers :

1. A,B 2. B,D 3. A,C 4. A,B
5. B,D,E 6. C,D,E 7. A,B,D,E 8. A,B,C,D,E
9. A,C,D,E 10. A,B,D 11. A

PGI 2003

1. **Prozone phenomenon is secondary syphilis is due to:**
A. Antigen excess
B. Antibody excess
C. False + reaction
D. False – reaction

2. **True about roseola infantum is:**
A. Also called 5th disease/6th disease
B. Caused by HSV 6, 7
C. Rash appears on the trunk, neck, buttocks
D. On defeverscence rash appears

3. **False about impetigo is:**
A. Mostly caused by staphylococcal or streptococcal or both
B. It predisposes to glomerulonephritis type 49, 55, 57, 66
C. Produces scar on healing
D. Erythromycin is drug of choice
E. It is infectious

4. **Fungal elements on skin scrapping or on section are seen in:**
A. Dermatophytosis
B. Chromomycosis
C. Mucomycosis
D. Histoplasmosis
E. Sporotrichosis

5. **True about acanthosis nigricans is:**
A. Most common seen in obesity
B. Seen in axilla
C. It signifies internal malignancy
D. It is associated with insulin resistance
E. Seen in old age

6. **Dermatophytosis are:**
A. T rubrum
B. T versicolor
C. Sporothrix
D. Microsporidium

7. **Secondary syphilis is manifested by:**
A. Painless lymphadenopathy
B. Pruritic rash
C. Mucosal erosion
D. Asymptomatic rash
E. Mostly asymptomatic

Answers :

1. B,D 2. B,C,D 3. B,CD 4. A,B
5. A,B,C,D 6. A 7. A,C,D,E

PGI 2002

1. **Isotretinoin is:**
A. Vitamin A analogue

B. Used in cystic acne
C. Safe in pregnancy
D. Use in psoriasis
E. Bony hyperostosis is a side effect

2. Wood's light is used for:
A. T capitis
B. Freckles
C. Vitiligo
D. Tuberous sclerosis

3. ANCA is seen:
A. WG
B. CSS
C. Microscopic polyangitis
D. Takayasu arteritis
E. SLE

4. Mucous lesions are seen in:
A. Secondary syphilis
B. DH
C. Psoriasis
D. Pemphigus
E. Porphyria

5. Predisposing factors for skin ca:
A. LP
B. Bowens
C. Psoriasis
D. Behcet's
E. UV rays

6. Regarding Fordyce's spots the following are true:
A. Ectopic sebaceous gland
B. Axilla
C. Healthy people
D. Are red

7. Zn deficiency results in:
A. Loss of libido
B. Poor weight gain
C. Poor wound healing
D. Sexual infantilism

8. Painful LN is seen in:
A. Donovaniosis
B. Syphilis
C. Chancroid
D. HSV
E. Gonorrhoea

9. PUVA therapy is used in:
A. Psoriasis
B. LP
C. Freckles
D. Melasma
E. Vitiligo

10. Mycobacterium causing skin ulcers:
A. M smegmatis
B. M scrofulaceum
C. M ulcerans
D. M fortuitium
E. M marinum

11. Cicatricial alopecia is seen in:
A. LP
B. DLE
C. Psoriasis
D. AA
E. SLE

Answers :

1. A,B,E	2. A,C,D	3. A,B,C	4. A,D
5. B,E	6. A,C	7. A, B, C	8. C, D
9. A, B, E	10. C	11. A, B	

PGI JUNE 2001

1. Staphylococcus can cause:
A. Echthyma
B. Erythrasma
C. Furuncle
D. Impetigo contagiosa
E. Sycosis barbae

2. Exacerbations of lesions in BB is seen in:
A. ENL
B. Lepra IR
C. JH reaction
D. Resolving reaction

3. Which of the following are photosensitive disease?
A. SLE
B. Liver spots
C. Calcinosis cutis
D. Morphoea
E. PCT

4. Skin hazards of swimming:
A. Verruca
B. PG
C. M marinum
D. M ulcerans

5. True about P alba:
A. No active treatment
B. Common in elderly
C. Variant of vitiligo
D. Common on the face
E. Presents as scaly macules

6. Skin test is done for which hypersensitive reactions?
A. Type I
B. Type II
C. Type III
D. Type IV

7. Which of the following is true of PRP?
A. Isolated patch of skin are seen
B. Cephalocaudal distribution
C. I.V. cyclosporine
D. Oral cyclosporine
E. Seen in females

Answers :

1. A,C,D,E	2. B	3. A,E	4. A,C
5. A,D,E	6. A,D	7. A,B,D	

PGI 2000

1. **Tinea capitis endothrix is caused by:**
   A. Epidermophyton B. T tonsurans
   C. T violaceum D. Microsporum
   E. T rubrum

2. **NF 2 is associated with:**
   A. Bilateral acoustic schwannoma
   B. Chromosome 22
   C. Lisch nodule
   D. Post subcapsular lenticular cataract

3. **Small vessel vasculitis is:**
   A. PAN
   B. Wegener's granulomatis
   C. Giant cell arteritis
   D. HSP
   E. CSS

4. **True about HSP:**
   A. Palpable purpura
   B. Kidney commonly affected
   C. C ANCA +
   D. Thrombocytopenia

5. **Features of secondary syphilis:**
   A. C acuminata
   B. C lata
   C. Mulberry molars
   D. Lesions over palm and sole

6. **True about keratoacanthoma:**
   A. Malignant like SCC
   B. Treatment same as for SCC
   C. Easy to differentiate from SCC histologically
   D. Treatment is by masterly inactivity

7. **Which of the following is a tuberculid?**
   A. L scrofulosorum B. L nitidus
   C. E nodosum D. L aureus

8. **Dyskeratosis is seen in:**
   A. Darier's B. P vulgaris
   C. Psoriasis D. Bowen disease
   E. Hailey-Hailey disease

9. **Eczema herpeticum is caused by:**
   A. HSV B. Varicella
   C. CMV D. HPV
   E. HSV 6

10. **Which of the following are pruritic?**
    A. L planus B. Sunburn
    C. Pemphigoid D. Psoriasis
    E. SLE

Answers :

1. B,C	2. A,B,D	3. B,D,E	4. A,B
5. B,D	6. D	7. A	8. A,D,E
9. A	10. A, B, C, D		

DPG 2009

1. **Necrotizing epitheloid cell granulomas are seen in all, *except:***
   A. Tuberculosis
   B. Wegener's granulomatosis
   C. Cat scratch disease
   D. Leprosy

2. **The skin changes seen in protein energy malnutrition can be due to deficiency of all the following nutrients, *except:***
   A. Zinc
   B. Tryptophan
   C. Essential fatty acids
   D. Pyridoxine

3. **Wavelength of Nd-Yag laser is:**
   A. 1064 nm
   B. 512 nm
   C. 594 nm
   D. 369 nm

4. **Intraepidermal blisters are seen in all of the following conditions, *except:***
   A. Pemphigus foliaceous
   B. Pemphigus vulgaris
   C. Paraneoplastic pemphigus
   D. Pemphigoid

5. **Following is a bacterial infection:**
   A. Pyoderma gangrenosum
   B. Impetigo herpetiformis
   C. Pitted keratolysis
   D. Mycosis fungoides

6. Following is a type of physical urticaria:

A. Dermographism
B. Urticaria pigmentosa
C. Urticaria vasculitis
D. Auto-immune urticaria

7. Which stage of syphilis is most contagious?

A. Primary B. Secondary
C. Early latent D. Late latent

8. Type-1 lepra reaction is commonly seen in:

A. Histoid leprosy
B. Lepromatous leprosy
C. Borderline tuberculoid leprosy
D. Polyneuritic leprosy

9. Photosensitivity is a feature of:

A. Porphyria cutanea tarda
B. Psoriasis
C. Pemphigoid
D. Pompholyx

10. Hypopigmented lesions are seen in:

A. Melasma
B. Pityriasis alba
C. Lichen planus pigmentosus
D. Urticaria pigmentosa

11. Potassium iodide is useful in the treatment of:

A. Sporotrichosis
B. Impetigo
C. Viral warts
D. Dermatitis herpetiformis

12. Which of the following tests is used for confirmation of diagnosis of contact dermatitis?

A. Intradermal test B. Patch test
C. Scratch test D. Prick test

13. Causative organisms for donovanosis is:

A. E. coli
B. Chlamydia trachomatis
C. H. ducreyi
D. Calymmatobacterium granulomatis

14. Keratoderma is a feature of:

A. Pityriasis rubra pilaris
B. Pemphigus
C. Pityriasis rosea
D. Psoriasis

15. Fixed drug eruptions can be seen more frequently with:

A. Penicillin B. Sulfonamide
C. Cetrizine D. Roxithromycin

16. The most common leukocytoclastic vasculitis affecting children is:

A. Takayasu disease
B. Mucocutaneous lymph node syndrome (Kawasaki disease)
C. Henoch-Schönlein purpura
D. Polyarteritis nodosa

17. Most common site of atopic dermatitis is:

A. Scalp B. Elbow
C. Trunk D. Anterior cubital fossa

18. An 8 years old boy from Bihar presents with a 6 months history of an ill defined, hypopigmented slightly atrophic macule on the face. The most likely diagnosis is:

A. Pityriasis alba
B. Indeterminate leprosy
C. Morphoea
D. Calcium deficiency

19. A 20-year-old male developed multiple tender non-indurated bleeding ulcers over prepuce 4 days after sexual exposure. The most probable diagnosis in this patient is:

A. Primary syphilis
B. Lymphogranuloma venerum
C. Chancroid
D. Donovanosis

20. Psoriasis is characterized by all, *except:*

A. Definite pink plaque with clear margin
B. In children disappear in 2 weeks to reappear again
C. Always associated with nail infection
D. Involves knees and elbow

21. Polygonal violaceous pruritic lesion is seen in:

A. Pityriasis rosea
B. Lichen planus
C. Psoriasis
D. Pemphigus vulgaris

22. Which naevi commonly predispose to malignant melanoma?

A. Dermal
B. Junctional
C. Congenital
D. Lentigo

23. Pruritis is seen in all, *except:*

A. Pemphigus
B. Lichen simplex chronicus
C. Psoriasis
D. Contact dermatitis

24. Pitting of nails is seen in:

A. Lichen planus
B. Psoriasis
C. Pemphigus
D. Arsenic poisoning

25. Chloroquine is used in the treatment of:

A. DLE
B. Pemphigus
C. Psoriasis
D. Nummular eczema

26. Herpes zoster is commonly seen in a:

A. Cervical region
B. Thoracic region
C. Lumbar region
D. Geniculate ganglion

27. Psoralen-A is used in the treatment of:

A. Pemphigus
B. Vitiligo
C. Pityriasis alba
D. Icthyosis

28. The most potent topical corticosteroids is:

A. Hydrocortisone butyrate cream 0.1%
B. Betamethasone valerate cream 0.5%
C. Clobetasol propionate cream 0.5%
D. Clobetasone butyrate cream 0.5%

29. Lepromatous leprosy shows all *except*:

A. Foamy macrophages
B. Masses of acid fast bacilli
C. Granulomas with epitheloid cells and giant cells
D. Lymph nodes may show foamy macrophages in the paracortical areas

30. Chiclero's ulcer is caused by:

A. Leishmania amazonensis
B. Leishmania braziliensis
C. Leishmania mexicane
D. Leishmania guyanensis

Answers :

1. C	2. D	3. A	4. D
5. A, C	6. A	7. B	8. C
9. A	10. B	11. A	12. B
13. D	14. A	15. B	16. C
17. D	18. B	19. C	20. C
21. B	22. C	23. A	24. B
25. A	26. B	27. B	28. C
29. C	30. C		

DPG 2007

1. Not a feature of Henoch-Schönlein purpura:

A. Purpura
B. Abdominal pain
C. Arthralgia
D. Seizures

2. Prick test is done to diagnose which hypersensitivity reaction?

A. Type 1
B. Type 2
C. Type 3
D. Type 4

3. PAN is associated with hepatitis:

A. A
B. B
C. C
D. D

4. Most common type of tuberculosis of skin is:

A. Lupus vulgaris
B. Scrofuloderma
C. Tuberculid
D. E indurativum

5. Scarring alopecia is seen in:

A. LE
B. AA
C. Pseudopelade
D. T effluvium

6. Miliaria is involvement of which glands?

A. Eccrine
B. Apocrine
C. Sebaceous
D. Endocrine

7. Normal commensal of sebaceous gland is:

A. P. acnes
B. S epidermis
C. S aureus
D. Candida

8. Most common site of mongolian spot is:

A. Face
B. Neck
C. Lumbosacral area
D. Chest

9. Not seen in leprosy:

A. Anesthetic patch
B. Nerve
C. Bullous
D. AFB

10. Patch test is used in:

A. Atopic dermatitis
B. Allergic contact dermatitis
C. Irritant contact dermatitis
D. Lichen simplex chronicus

11. Hemangioma in a ten-year-old boy on the tongue which is symptomatic is best treated by:

A. Wait and watch
B. Radiotherapy
C. Surgery
D. Laser

Answers :

1. D	2. A	3. B	4. A
5. C	6. A	7. A	8. C
9. C	10. B	11. C	

UPSC 2009

1. Regarding measles, which one of the following statements is not correct?

A. It is caused by paramyxo virus infection
B. Rash is usually vesicular
C. Infection spreads by droplets
D. Incubation period is 14 days

2. Secondary syphilis is characterized by the following *except:*

A. Occurs 6-8 weeks after development of chancre
B. Painful and itchy maculopapular lesions
C. Constitutional features are present
D. Meningitis, hepatitis, glomerulonephritis and uveitis may occur

3. In an immunocompromised patient with local gumma like tumors and granulomatous lesions of lungs, bones, brain and meninges, the most likely diagnosis is:

A. Tuberculosis
B. Leprosy
C. Sarcoidosis
D. Cryptococcosis

4. Which one of the following is not a fungal infection?

A. Chromomycosis
B. Pheohyphomycosis
C. Actinomycosis
D. Blastomycosis

5. With regard to vitiligo, which one of the following is not correct?

A. Generalized vitiligo is often symmetrical
B. Trauma and sunburn may precipitate vitiligo
C. It is a congenital condition
D. Focal areas of melanocyte loss are observed

6. The following diseases are characterized by bullous eruptions, *except:*

A. Porphyria cutanea tarda
B. Variegate porphyria
C. Dermatitis herpetiformis
D. Lichen planus

7. Which one of the following features differentiates lepromatous leprosy from tuberculoid leprosy?

A. Absence of infectivity of affected patients
B. Organisms are scanty in number
C. Blood-borne spread from the dermis throughout the body
D. Anaesthetic hypopigmented skin macules and plaques

8. Recurrent painful orogenital ulcers with arthritis is most likely due to:

A. Gonorrhea
B. Syphilis
C. Reiter's syndrome
D. Behcet's syndrome

9. Which one of the following is a characteristic feature of drug induced lupus?

A. Antihistone antibodies
B. Anti Ro antibodies
C. Anti La antibodies
D. Anti ds DNA antibodies

Answers :

1. B	2. B	3. A	4. C
5. C	6. D	7. D	8. D
9. A			

UPSC 2008

1. All are seen in lepromatous leprosy *except:*

A. Type 2 reaction
B. Inflammatory reaction is sparse
C. Loss of sensation occurs late
D. Surface of the skin lesions is smooth and shiny

2. The following are the stigmata of syphilis, *except:*

A. Hutchinson incisors
B. Saddle nose
C. AR
D. Sabre tibia

3. Causes of pruritus in 3rd trimester are all *except:*

A. Prurigo gestationis

B. Obsteric cholestasis
C. Pemphigoid gestationis
D. Pruritic folliculitis

4. Which of the following is not seen in pellagra?

A. It is seen in carcinoid syndrome
B. Diarrhoea and dementia are common
C. Casal necklace may be seen
D. Response to niacin is slow

5. All can cause bullous lesions, *except:*

A. Pemphigus
B. Impetigo
C. TEN
D. P rosea

6. Nikolsky sign is characteristic of:

A. TEN
B. Psoriasis
C. Darier's disease
D. Pemphigus

7. A 45 years old female has headache with a cord like structure on the scalp with raised ESR, what is it?

A. Tension headache
B. Migraine
C. Temporal arteritis
D. TB meningitis

8. Which of the following are to be avoided in a patient of dermatitis herpetiformis?

A. Bread
B. Noodles
C. Dosa
D. Atta

9. Which of the following is not a feature of Henoch-Schönlein purpura?

A. Polyarthalgia
B. Cure by steroids
C. Hematuria
D. Abdominal pain

10. Which of the following does not cause small vessel vasculitis?

A. Churg-Strauss syndrome
B. Henoch-Schönlein purpura
C. Kawasaki disease
D. Microscopic polyangitis

Answers :

1. B	2. C	3. D	4. D
5. D	6. D	7. C	8. D
9. B	10. C		

Part VI

Test Series

This should be done before taking any exam.

TEST 1

1. By when is FTA-ABS test positive in syphilis?

A. 1 week B. 3 days
C. 2 weeks D. 4 days

2. A 30 years old male had severely itchy papula vesicular lesions on extremities, knees, elbows and buttocks for one year. Direct immunofluorescence staining of the lesions showed IgA deposition at dermoepidermal junction. The most probable diagnosis is:

A. Pemphigus vulgaris
B. Bullous pemphigoid
C. Dermatitis herpetiformis
D. Nummular eczema

3. A 5-year-old male child has multiple hyper-pigmented macules over the trunk, on rubbing the lesion with the rounded end of a pen. He developed urticarial wheal, confined to the border of the lesion. The most likely diagnosis is:

A. Fixed drug eruption B. Lichen planus
C. Urticaria pigmentosa D. Urticarial vasculitis

4. A 25-year-old man presents with recurrent episodes of flexural eczema contact, recurrent skin infections and severe abnormal cramps and diarrhea upon taking sea foods. He is suffering from:

A. Seborrheic dermatitis
B. Atopic dermatitis
C. Airborne contact dermatitis
D. Nummular dermatitis

5. Tinea capitis that is Wood's lamp negative and is characterized by scutulae is caused by:

A. T schoenleinii
B. Microsporum audouinii
C. Microsporum canis
D. Trichophyton tonsurans

6. Coral red fluorescence Wood's lamp seen in:

A. Porphyria cutanea tarda
B. Hypomelanosis
C. Livedo reticularis
D. Erythrasma

7. A boy aged 8 from Tamil Nadu has a white non-anesthetic, scaly hypopigmented macule on his face:

A. Pityriasis alba
B. Indeterminate leprosy
C. Pityriasis versicolor
D. Pure neuritic leprosy

8. "Oil drop" phenomenon is seen in:

A. Clubbing
B. Psoriasis of nails
C. Lichen planus of nails
D. Tinea unguium

9. Munro's microabscesses are seen in:

A. Stratum granulosum B. Stratum corneum
C. Basal layer D. Papillary tips

10. In pustular psoriasis, the treatment of choice is:

A. Acitretin
B. Methotrexate
C. Systemic corticosteroids
D. Psoralen + UV therapy

11. For erythrodermic psoriasis the treatment of choice is:

A. Topical corticosteroids B. Coal tar topically
C. Methotrexate D. Corticosteroids

12. Tinea "incognito" is due to inappropriate use of systemic and topical:

A. Antibiotics B. Antifungals
C. Steroids D. Antivirals

13. Causative agent of tinea versicolor is:

A. Tinea schoenleinii
B. Tinea rubrum
C. Malassezia furfur
D. Epidermophyton floccosum

14. Fordyce spots are ectopic:

A. Mucosal glands B. Apocrine glands
C. Eccrine glands D. Sebaceous glands

15. HLA strongly associated with psoriasis is:

A. HLAA5 B. HLA B27
C. HLA B8 D. HLA Cw6

16. Berloque dermatitis is due to contact with which of the following?

A. Plants B. Food
C. Cosmetics D. Metal

17. Growing phase of hair is:

A. Catagen and telogen B. Telogen
C. Anagen D. Catagen

18. Pseudopelade is also known as:

A. Cicatricial alopecia
B. Traction alopecia
C. Premature alopecia
D. Alopecia totalis

19. Not a characteristic feature of Melkersson-Rosenthal syndrome:

A. Plication of tongue
B. Black hairy tongue
C. Labial edema
D. Recurrent VII nerve palsy

20. Most severe form of scabies is:

A. Norwegian scabies B. Nodular scabies
C. Animal scabies D. Genital scabies

21. Permethrin is useful in:

A. Leishmaniasis B. Body louse
C. Leprosy D. Scabies

22. "Cradle cap" is a special form of:

A. Down's syndrome
B. Cephalhematoma
C. Seborrheic dermatitis
D. Alopecia steatoides

23. Most sensitive index to assess the drug effectiveness in skin smears of leprosy patient is:

A. Culture of lesion
B. Granuloma index
C. Morphological index
D. Bacteriological index

24. Maximum suppression of cell mediated immunity occurs in:

A. Indeterminate leprosy
B. Tuberculoid leprosy
C. Lepromatous leprosy
D. Borderline leprosy

25. Skin pigmentation is a side effect of:

A. Steroid
B. Dapsone
C. Clofazimine
D. Rifampicin

26. Dose of dapsone is:

A. 1-2 mg/kg B. 5 mg/kg
C. 10 mg/kg D. 20 mg/kg

27. Daily dose of thalidomide for controlling ENL is:

A. 100 mg B. 200-400 mg
C. 500 mg D. 1000 mg only

28. Drug of choice in type I lepra reaction with severe neuritis is:

A. Chloroquine B. Thalidomide
C. Clofazimine D. Systemic steroid

29. Ichthyosis vulgaris is inherited as:

A. X-linked recessive
B. X-linked dominant
C. Autosomal recessive
D. Autosomal dominant

30. Ichthyosis is associated with all, *except*:

A. Lymphogranuloma venereum
B. Hypothyroidism
C. Hodgkin's disease
D. AIDS

31. Dhobi itch is:

A. Tinea versicolor B. Tinea capitis
C. Tinea barbae D. Tinea cruris

32. Rhinophyma is:

A. Glandular form of acne rosacea
B. Form of acne vulgaris
C. Affects the scalp
D. A form of dermatofibroma

33. For pediculosis corporis the treatment of choice is:

A. Disinfection of clothes
B. Four applications of benzyl benzoate
C. One application of benzyl benzoate
D. Three applications of gamma benzene hexachloride

34. Crystalline miliaria occurs due to obstruction of:

A. Accessory sweat gland
B. Hair roots
C. Sweat glands
D. Sebaceous glands

35. Most common site of herpes gestationis:

A. Infraorbital
B. Periumbilical region

C. Thorax
D. Vulva

36. Not a skin manifestation of secondary syphilis:
A. Vesicle
B. Pustular syphilides
C. Papule
D. Bilaterally symmetrical

37. Yaws is caused by:
A. Treponema pallidum
B. Treponema pertenue
C. Treponema carateum
D. Treponema endemicum

38. In which of the following condition, intraepidermal blisters are seen:
A. Pemphigus foliaceus
B. PCT
C. Dermatitis herpetiformis
D. Erythema marginatum

39. A child presents with slapped cheek appearance of face, diagnosis is:
A. Pityriasis alba
B. Leprosy
C. Tinea versicolor
D. Erythema infectiosum

40. Chloroquine is used in treatment of:
A. Discoid lupus erythematosus
B. Lichen planus
C. Psoriasis
D. Pemphigoid

41. Tzanck cell is a:
A. Lymphocyte B. Monocyte
C. Neutrophil D. Keratinocyte

42. Underlying internal malignancy is shown by all, *except:*
A. Erythema gyratum repens
B. Bullous pemphigoid
C. Bullous pyoderma
D. Acanthosis nigricans

43. Lagophthalmos is seen in:
A. Leprosy B. Syphilis
C. Peripheral neuritis D. HZV infection

44. Dyskeratosis is a feature of:
A. Darier's disease
B. Pemphigus vulgaris
C. Psoriasis
D. Lichen planus

45. Tzanck smear in a patient of bullous lesions shows:
A. Absence of melanin pigment
B. Leukocytosis
C. Acantholysis
D. Langerhans' cells

46. Darier's sign is seen in:
A. Xeroderma pigmentosa
B. Urticaria pigmentosa
C. Herpes zoster
D. Glucagonoma

47. Drug of choice in a male with androgenic alopecia:
A. Minoxidil 2%
B. Finasteride 1 mg
C. Cyproterone acetate
D. Finasteride 2 mg

48. Gonococcus is:
A. Extracellular gram-positive
B. Intracytoplasmic gram positive
C. Intracellular gram negative
D. Intranuclear gram positive

49. In gonorrhea the drug of choice is:
A. Benzyl penicillin
B. Phenoxymethyl penicillin
C. Ceftriaxone
D. Benzathine penicillin

50. Treatment with griseofulvin in fungal infection of the finger nails is for:
A. 6 weeks B. 4 weeks
C. 2 months D. 3 months

51. Reliable test for chancroid detection:
A. Skin test B. Biopsy
C. Culture D. Clinical examination

52. Lisch nodules are seen in:
A. Albright's syndrome
B. Neurofibromatosis
C. Tuberous sclerosis
D. Piebaldism

53. Ocular hallmark of pseudoxanthoma elasticum is:
A. Retinal hemorrhage B. Iritis
C. Angioid streak D. Keratitis

54. Porphyria cutanea tarda can be treated by:
A. High dose of systemic steroids
B. Hemoglobin
C. Low dose chloroquine
D. Metronidazole

55. Quincke's disease is popularly known as:
A. Norwegian scabies
B. Angioneurotic edema
C. Seborrheic dermatitis
D. Saddle nose

56. The test likely to help in diagnosis of a patient who presents with an itchy annular plaque on the face is:
A. Gram's stain
B. Potassium hydroxide mount
C. Tissue smear
D. Wood's lamp examination

57. In a fair patient early diagnosis of vitiligo is by:
A. Luminol spray
B. Infrared photography
C. Ultraviolet light
D. Magnifying lens

58. Castellani's paint contains all of the following, *except:*
A. Basic fuchsin B. Phenol
C. Benzene hexachloride D. Boric acid

59. Erythrasma is caused by:
A. Corynebacterium minutissimum
B. Corynebacterium diphtheriae
C. Corynebacterium vaginalis
D. Corynebacterium ulcerans

60. In a patch of vitiligo when the hair is white it is called:
A. Heterochromia B. Poliosis
C. Tiger tail D. Leukotrichia

61. The treatment of choice of Sweet syndrome is:
A. Antibiotic B. Antifungals
C. Corticosteroids D. UV light

62. Ciclopirox olamine is used in:
A. Dermatophytosis B. Psoriasis
C. Acne **D.** Lichen planus

63. Crocodile skin or phrynoderma is seen in:
A. Toxic epidermal necrolysis
B. Darier's syndrome
C. Psoriasis
D. Vitamin A deficiency

64. Cells cultured from patients with this disorder exhibit low activity for the nucleotide excision repair process. This autosomal recessive genetic disease includes marked sensitivity to sunlight, ultraviolet light, with subsequent formation of multiple skin cancer and premature death, the disorder is:
A. Acute intermittent porphyria
B. Xeroderma pigmentosa
C. Ataxia telangiectasia
D. Alkaptonuria

65. Meirwosky phenomenon is because of which form of UV radiation (immediate pigment darkening):
A. UV-B B. UV-A
C. UV-C D. None

66. "Black dot" ring worm is caused by:
A. Microsporum B. Epidermophyton
C. Candida D. Trichophyton

67. Which of the following are premalignant conditions of skin?
A. Bowen's disease B. Actinic keratosis
C. Both D. None

68. Suprabasal blister is a characteristic feature of:
A. Insect bite B. Pemphigoid
C. Herpes zoster D. Pemphigus

69. Pruritus is not seen in:
A. Contact dermatitis
B. Psoriasis
C. Pemphigus
D. Lichen simplex chronicus

70. Rarest variety of pemphigus which is also associated with SLE is:
A. Pemphigus vulgaris
B. Pemphigus erythematosis/senear usher syndrome
C. Pemphigus foliaceus
D. Pemphigus vegetans

71. False about pityriasis alba:

A. No active treatment required
B. Common in children
C. Variant of vitiligo
D. Common over the face

72. Arvinder, a 24-year-old woman, presents with multiple erythematous annular lesions with collarette scales predominantly arranged over the trunk. The most likely diagnosis is:

A. Pityriasis rosea
B. Pityriasis rubra pilaris
C. Pityriasis versicolor
D. Pityriasis lichenoid chronica

73. A 32-year-old male, Kallu, who recently visited a seacoast, presented with an ulcer over the left leg. The probable cause is:

A. Pasteurella multocida
B. Micrococcus catarrhalis
C. Vibrio vulnificus
D. Neisseria catarrhalis

74. A patient gets recurrent urticaria while doing exercising and on exposure to sunlight. Which of the following is the most likely cause?

A. Cholinergic urticaria
B. Chronic idiopathic urticaria
C. Universal dermographism
D. Pressure urticaria

75. Koenen's periungual fibromas are seen in >50% of cases of:

A. Tuberous sclerosis
B. Sturge-Weber syndrome
C. Ataxia telangiectasia
D. Neurofibromatosis

76. Haemophilus ducreyi is the causative agent of:

A. Hard chancre
B. Urethritis
C. Soft sore
D. Granuloma inguinale

77. Nail involvement is not a feature of:

A. Eczema
B. DLE
C. Psoriasis
D. Lichen planus

78. A 30-year-old male had severely itchy bullous lesions on trunk for one year. Direct immunofluorescence staining of the lesions showed IgG deposition at dermoepidermal junction. The most probable diagnosis is:

A. Pemphigus vulgaris
B. Bullous pemphigoid
C. Dermatitis herpetiformis
D. Nummular eczema

79. Maculae ceruleae are caused by:

A. Pubic lice
B. Head lice
C. Body lice
D. Mites

80. Which of the following diagnoses active infection in syphilis?

A. VDRL 1:8
B. IgM –FTA-ABS
C. TPHA
D. VDRL 1:4

81. A 12-year-old boy from Rajasthan had a gradually progressive plaque on a buttock for the last 3 years. The plaque was 15 cm in diameter, annular in shape, with crusting and indurations at the periphery and scarring at the center. The most likely diagnosis is:

A. Tinea corporis
B. Granuloma annulare
C. Leishmaniasis
D. Borderline leprosy

82. A 22-year-old woman developed small itchy wheals after physical exertion, walking in the sun, eating hot spicy food and when she was angry. The most likely diagnosis is:

A. Cholinergic urticaria
B. Solar urticaria
C. Heat urticaria
D. Chronic idiopathic urticaria

83. A 45-year-old male had multiple hypoanesthetic mildly erythematous large plaques with elevated margins on trunk and extremities. His ulnar and lateral popliteal nerves on both sides were enlarged. The most probable diagnosis is:

A. Lepromatous leprosy
B. Borderline leprosy
C. Borderline tuberculoid leprosy
D. Borderline lepromatous leprosy

84. A 6-month-old infant presented with multiple papules and exudative lesions on the face, scalp, trunk and few vesicles on the palms and soles for 2 weeks. His mother had history of itchy lesions. The most likely diagnosis is:

A. Scabies

B. Infantile eczema
C. Infantile seborrheic dermatitis
D. Impetigo contagiosa

85. A 10-year-old schoolgirl has recurrent episodes of boils on the scalp. The boils subside with antibiotic therapy but recur after some time. The most likely cause of the recurrences is:

A. Primary immunodeficiency syndrome
B. Juvenile diabetes mellitus
C. Pediculus capitis
D. HIV infection

86. A 40-year-old man had multiple blisters over the trunk and extremities. Direct immunofluorescence studies showed IgG. Localized to upper epidermis which of the following is the most likely diagnosis?

A. Pemphigus vulgaris
B. Pemphigus foliaceus
C. Bullous pemphigoid
D. Dermatitis herpetiformis

87. A 40-year-old woman presented with an 8 months history of erythema and swelling of the periorbital region and papules and plaques on the dorsolateral aspect of forearms and knuckles with ragged cuticles. There was no muscle weakness. The most likely diagnosis is:

A. SLE
B. Dermatomyositis
C. Systemic sclerosis
D. Mixed connective tissue disorder

88. A 56-year-old man has painful weeping rashes over the upper eyelid and forehead for the last two days along with ipsilateral acute punctate keratopathy. One year back, he had chemotherapy for non-Hodgkin's lymphoma. There is no other abnormality. Which of the following is the most likely diagnosis?

A. Impetigo
B. SLE
C. Herpes zoster
D. Pyoderma gangrenosum

89. A 36-year-old sexually active male presented with asymptomatic multiple, erythematosus, annular lesions with a collarette of scales at the periphery of the lesions present on the trunk, the most likely diagnosis is:

A. Pityriasis versicolor
B. Pityriasis alba
C. Secondary syphilis
D. Pityriasis rubra pilaris

90. A 40-year-old woman presents with a 2 years history of erythematosus papulopustular lesions on the convexities of the face. There is a background of erythema and telangiectasia. The most likely diagnosis in this patient is:

A. Acne vulgaris
B. Acne rosacea
C. Systemic lupus erythematosus
D. Polymorphic light eruption

91. An 8-year-old boy from Bihar presents with a 6 months history of an ill-defined hypopigmented slightly atrophic macule on the face. The most likely diagnosis is:

A. Pityriasis alba
B. Indeterminate leprosy
C. Morphea
D. Calcium deficiency

92. A 27-year-old sexually active male develops a vesiculobullous lesion on the glans soon after taking tablet paracetamol for fever. The lesion healed with hyperpigmentation. The most likely diagnosis is:

A. Behçet's syndrome
B. Herpes genitalis
C. Fixed drug eruption
D. Pemphigus vulgaris

93. Which of the following drugs are effective in the treatment of pityriasis versicolor, and is fungicidal?

A. Selenium disulphide
B. Ketoconazole
C. Terbinafine
D. Clotrimazole

94. A 36-year-old factory worker developed non-itchy, annular scaly plaques in both groins. Application of a corticosteroid ointment led to temporary relief but the plaques continued to extend at the periphery. The most likely diagnosis is:

A. Erythema annulare centrifugum
B. Tinea cruris
C. Annular lichen planus
D. Tinea incognito

Answers :

1. A	2. C	3. C	4. B
5. A	6. D	7. A	8. B
9. B	10. A	11. C	12. C
13. C	14. D	15. D	16. C
17. C	18. A	19. B	20. A
21. D	22. C	23. C	24. C
25. C	26. A	27. B	28. D
29. D	30. A	31. D	32. A
33. A	34. C	35. B	36. A
37. B	38. A	39. D	40. A
41. D	42. C	43. A,D	44. A
45. C	46. B	47. B	48. C
49. C	50. D	51. C	52. B
53. C	54. C	55. B	56. B
57. C	58. C	59. A	60. D
61. C	62. A	63. D	64. B
65. B	66. D	67. C	68. D
69. C	70. B	71. C	72. A
73. C	74. A	75. A	76. C
77. B	78. B	79. A	80. B
81. C	82. A	83. C	84. A
85. C	86. B	87. B	88. C
89. C	90. B	91. B	92. C
93. C	94. D		

TEST 2

1. **Which of the following statements about lepromin test is not true?**
   A. It is negative in most children in first 6 months of life
   B. It is a diagnostic test
   C. It is an important aid to classify type of leprosy disease
   D. It assess CMI

2. **Anagen phase of the hair indicates:**
   A. The phase of activity and growth
   B. The phase of transition
   C. The phase of resting
   D. The phase of degeneration

3. **'Chancre redux' is a clinical feature of:**
   A. Early relapsing syphilis
   B. Late syphilis
   C. Chancroid
   D. Recurrent herpes simplex infection

4. **Max Joseph's space is a histopathological feature of:**
   A. Psoriasis vulgaris B. Lichen planus
   C. Pityriasis rosea D. Parapsoriasis

5. **Ivermectin is indicated in the treatment of:**
   A. Syphilis B. Scabies
   C. Tuberculosis D. Dermatophytosis

6. **The main cytokine, involved in erythema nodosum leprosum (ENL) reaction, is:**
   A. Interleukin-2
   B. Interferon-gamma
   C. Tumor necrosis factor-alpha
   D Macrophage colony stimulating factor

7. **The following drug is not used for the treatment of type II lepra reaction:**
   A. Chloroquin B. Thalidomide
   C. Cyclosporine D. Corticosteroids

8. **The following test is not used for diagnosis of leprosy:**
   A. Lepromin test
   B. Slit skin smear
   C. Fine needle aspiration cytology
   D. Skin biopsy

9. **Air-borne contact dermatitis can be diagnosed by:**
   A. Skin biopsy
   B. Patch test
   C. Prick test
   D. Estimation of serum IgE levels

10. **A patient with HIV disease is on Highly Active Anti-Retroviral Therapy (HAART). He develops tuberculosis. Which one of the following anti-tubercular drugs interferes with HAART?**
    A. Isoniazid B. Ethambutol
    C. Pyrazinamide D. Rifampicin

11. **Which one of the following is the drug of choice for treating systemic fungal infection?**
    A. Griseofulvin B. Amphotericin B
    C. Ketoconazole D. Co-trimoxazole

12. **A 35-year-old alcoholic presents with diarrhoea and scaly rash on his neck, hands and feet. He will improve if he is treated with which one of the following?**
    A. Vitamin A B. Thiamine
    C. Folic acid D. Nicotinic acid

13. **Consider the following regarding a melanotic melanoma *except*:**
    A. Non pigmented and appearing as ink or flesh coloured
    B. Characterized by a radial growth phase
    C. Inability of these poorly differentiated cancer cells to synthesize melanin pigment
    D. Precursor lesion is usually lentigo maligna

14. **Which of the above are correct regarding leprosy?**
    A. Neuritic leprosy is very common
    B. BI > 2 + is mB leprosy
    C. BI = 1+ is mB leprosy
    D. Surgery is the best option of Nx abscess

15. **Which one of the following pairs is not correctly matched?**
    A. Acantholysis: P. vulgaris
    B. Hypopigmented: Leprosy anaesthetic patch
    C. Vesiculobullous: Secondary syphilis lesions
    D. Kaposi's sarcoma: AIDS

16. **What is the cutaneous viral infection which is commonly seen in children and characterized by single or multiple pearly-white skin coloured smooth dome shaped papules with central pitting?**

A. Chicken pox
B. Small pox
C. Molluscum contagiosum
D. Verruca vulgaris

17. Wegener's granulomatosis is characterised by the following *except:*

A. Vasculitis of respiratory tract
B. Granulomatous uveitis
C. Granulomatous hepatitis
D. Glomerulonephritis

18. A VDRL reactive mother gave birth to an infant. All of the following would help in determining the risk of transmission to the infant *except*:

A. TPHA test on the serum sample of the mother
B. TPHA test on the serum sample of the infant
C. VDRL on the paired serum sample of the infant and mother
D. Time interval between the treatment of the mother and her delivery

19. A 6-month-old infant had itchy erythematous papules and exudative lesions on the scalp, face, groins and axillae for one month. She also had vesicular lesions on the palms. The most likely diagnosis is:

A. Congenital syphilis
B. Seborrheic dermatitis
C. Scabies
D. Psoriasis

20. Pterygium of nail is characteristically seen in:

A. Lichen planus
B. Psoriasis
C. Tinea unguium
D. Alopecia areata

21. A patient had seven irregular hyperpigmented macules on the trunk and multiple small hyperpigmented macules in the axillae and groins since early childhood. There were no other skin lesions. Which is the most likely investigation to support the diagnosis?

A. Slit lamp examination of eye
B. Measurement of intraocular tension
C. Examination of fundus
D. Retinal artery angiography

22. A 24-year-old unmarried woman has multiple nodular, cystic, pustular and comedonic lesions on face, upper back and shoulders for 2 years. The drug of choice for her treatment would be:

A. Acitretin
B. Isotretinoin
C. Doxycycline
D. Azithromycin

23. A 45-year-old farmer has itchy erythematous papular lesions on face, neck, V area of chest, dorsum of hands and forearms for 3 years. The lesions are more severe in summers and improve by 75% in winters. The most appropriate test to diagnose the condition would be:

A. Skin biopsy
B. Estimation of IgE levels in blood
C. Patch test
D. Intradermal prick test

24. Anticentromere antibodies are most commonly associated with:

A. Diffuse cutaneous systemic sclerosis
B. Mixed connective tissue disease
C. CREST syndrome
D. Polymyositis

25. A 40 years old woman presented to the gynecologist with complaints of profuse vaginal discharge. There was no discharge from the cervical os on the speculum examination. The diagnosis of bacterial vaginosis was made based upon all of the following findings on microscopy, *except:*

A. Abundance of gram variable coccobacilli
B Absence of lactobacilli
C. Abundance of polymorphs
D. Presence of clue cells

26. Drug induced lupus can be identified by:

A. Anti-histone antibodies
B. Double stranded DNA antibodies
C. Antinuclear antibodies
D. Anti-SM antibodies

27. An adult man comes with urethral discharge the gram stain is negative, what medium should be used for culture?

A. Mc coy cell
B. Blood agar
C. Choclate agar
D. Cetrimide agar

28. A diagnosed case of BT with neuritis is treated by:

A. MDT
B. MDT and steroids
C. Steroids
D. MDT and aspirin

29. Leprosy effects all, *except:*

A. Uterus
B. Ovary
C. Eye
D. Nerve

30. All are true about Raynaud's diseases *except:*

A. Good prognosis
B. More in females
C. ANA test is positive
D. Raynaud's phenomenon is common presentation

31. Finasteride acts by:

A. Alpha blockade
B. 5 alpha reductase
C. Selective alpha blockade
D. Acts by blocking androgen

32. Which of the following about mycoses fungoides is not true?

A. It is the most common skin lymphoma
B. Pautriers microabscess are common
C. It has an indolent course and good prognosis
D. It presents with diffuse erythroderma

33. In acute graft versus host disease which of the following organs are not affected?

A. Skin B. Lung
C. Liver D. Kidney

34. A 22 years old female comes with a history of ingestion of groundnuts followed by swelling of tongue and respiratory distress. What is the possible cause?

A. Angioedema
B. Periapical abscess
C. Foreign body bronchus
D. Foreign body larynx

35. A infant presented with non-itchy vesicles and bulla on hands and feet at birth. Which of the following investigations will you perform?

A. Paired VDRL samplers of infant and mother
B. VDRL of mother
C. Biopsy
D. TPHA of infant

36. What is the cause of half half nail in renal failure?

A. Defect in keratin
B. Defect in collagen
C. Defect in vasculature
D. Chronic itch

37. A 45-year-old male comes with painful persistent oral erosions with flaccid bulla on the trunk, what is the most likely diagnosis?

A. Bullous pemphigoid
B. Pemphigus vulgaris
C. Erythema multiforme
D. Cicatricial pemphigoid

38. Which of the following is seen in Hailey-Hailey disease?

A. Row of tombstones
B. Subepidermal bulla
C. DIF showing IgG
D. Dilapidated brick wall appearance

39. Inverted saucer lesions is seen in:

A. BT **B.** BB
C. BL **D.** BL in reaction

40. Which of the following is diagnostic for Langerhan cell histiocytosis?

A. CD1 a
B. S 100
C. Peanut agglutinin
D. Thromobocytopenia

41. A child comes with a congenital dermatomal hypopigmentation which disappears on diascopy test?

A. Vitiligo
B. Nevus depigmentosus
C. Nevus anaemicus
D. Hypomelanosis of ito

42. Which of the following is a drug of choice for psoriatic arthritis?

A. Retinoids B. Methotrexate
C. Cyclosporine D. Etanercept

43. Which of the following is a cause of kerion?

A. T rubrum B. T tonsurans
C. M canis D. T mentagrophytes

44. Which of the following drugs are useless in P versicolor?

A. Itraconazole B. Topical terbinafine
C. Griseofulvin D. Fluconazole

45. Oral hairy leukoplakia is caused by:

A. HSV 1 B. HSV 7
C. HSV 3 D. HSV 4

46. Which of the following antibodies are associated with renal nephritis in SLE?

A. ANA B. Ds DNA
C. Anti SM D. Oral ulcers

47. Which of the following is diagnostic of dermatomyositis?

A. Heliotrope rash B. Gottron's papules
C. Calcinosis cutis D. Muscle weakness

48. Pityriasis rosea is a:

A. Chronic relapsing disease
B. Caused by dermatophyte
C. It is an autoimmune disease
D. Self resolving

49. Which of the following can be depressed?

A. Plaque B. Macule
C. Nodule D. Papule

50. Thimble pitting of nails is seen in:

A. Alopecia areata
B. Lichen planus
C. Pityriasis rubra pilaris
D. Pityriasis rosea

51. A man aged 30 years presents with alopecia, boggy scalp swelling and easily pluckable hair. Next step in establishing diagnosis would be:

A. KOH smear B. Culture sensitivity
C. Biopsy D. A + B

52. Child presented with overnight rash all over body. Two weeks ago he had an episode of abdominal pain. There was mild pallor and no hepatosplenomegaly. What is the likely diagnosis?

A. Aplastic anaemia
B. ITP
C. Acute leukemia
D. Acute post viral syndrome

53. Child presented with *petechial* rash all over body with *ecchymosis* on the lower limb. Two weeks ago he had an episode of *abdominal pain*. There was *severe pallor*, weakness and no *hepatosplenomegaly*. What is the likely diagnosis?

A. Aplastic anaemia
B. ITP
C. Acute leukemia
D. Acute post viral syndrome

54. A 7-year-old child presents with fever, given cefaclor for 8 days out of 10 days, presents with rash, pruritus, lymphadenopathy. What is the diagnosis?

A. Kawasaki syndrome
B. Half treated meningitis
C. Inf. mononucleosis
D. Hypersensitivity reaction

55. A premature LBW baby, presented with a bullous rash at birth and on X-ray there was periostitis. What is the next investigation?

A. VDRL of mother and child
B. ELISA–HIV
C. PCR Tb
D. Hbsag of mother

56. FK 506 is a drug used in vitiligo and atopic dermatitis, it is a:

A. Macrolide antibiotic
B. Immunoglobulin
C. Muscle relaxant
D. Opioid analgesic

57. Which of the following conditions show the Michaelis Guttman Body:

A. Malakoplakia
B. Rhinoscleroma
C. Botyromycosis
D. TB

Answers :

1. B	2. A	3. A	4. B
5. B	6. C	7. C	8. C
9. B	10. D	11. B	12. D
13. B,D	14. C	15. C	16. C
17. C	18. B	19. C	20. A
21. A	22. B	23. C	24. C
25. C	26. A	27. A	28. B
29. B	30. C	31. B	32. C
33. D	34. A	35. A	36. C
37. B	38. D	39. D	40. C
41. C	42. D	43. D	44. C
45. D	46. B	47. B	48. D
49. A	50. A	51. D	52. D
53. A	54. D	55. A	56. A
57. A			

TEST 3

1. A child comes in summers with itchy papules on the limb and trunk, what is the probable diagnosis?
A. Photodermatitis B. Contact dermatitis
C. PCT D. Papular urticaria

2. In which type of leprosy Swiss cheese lesions are seen?
A. BT B. BL
C. BB D. LL

3. Which of the follwing is always BI (-)?
A. Be B. LL
C. TT D. Neuritic Hansen

4. Which of the following drugs are not useful in type II lepra reactions?
A. Thalidomide B. Cyclosporine
C. Chloroquine D. Steroids

5. What is the time required for the MI of a patient on treatment to become –0 on MDT?
A. 6 weeks B. 6 months
C. 1 year D. 2 years

6. In which form of leprosy is the lepromin (-ve)?
A. TT B. BB
C. IL D. BT

7. Which is the most common cranial nerve to be affected in leprosy?
A. II B. III
C. V D. VII

8. A case with bilateral inguinal swelling comes to the STD clinic what organism will you provisionally treat?
A. LGV and chancroid
B. LGV and HSV
C. Chancroid and syphilis
D. Gonorrhoea and syphilis

9. In an HIV positive patient of syphilis what treatment will you give in early syphilis?
A. Benzathine penicillin G, 2.4 million units IM
B. Benzathine penicillin G, 2.4 million units IM one dose weekly for three weeks
C. Doxycycline, 100 mg PO, twice daily for 15 days
D. Doxycycline, 100 mg PO, twice daily for 30 days

10. A case of urethral discharge comes and the smear shows ICDC with PMN. How will you treat this case?
A. Azithromycin 2 G stat
B. Doxycycline 100 mg orally twice a day for 7 days
C. Ciprofloxacin 50 mg BD for 7 days
D. Plenty of fluids

11. How will you treat a case of chancroid with HIV?
A. Azithromycin 2 G stat
B. Doxycycline 100 mg orally twice a day for 7 days
C. Ciprofloxacin 50 mg BD for 7 days
D. Erythromycin 500 mg QID for 7 days

12. Which of the following type of psoriasis can be treated by antibiotics?
A. Pustular B. Erythrodermic
C. Guttate D. Inverse

13. Salt split method is used to diagnose which one of the following?
A. Pemphigus B. Miliaria
C. Herpes D. Bullous pemphigoid

14. Which of the following is not an autoimmune disorder?
A. Pemphigus
B. Bullous pemphigoid
C. Cong EB
D. Herpes gestationis

15. Pediculosis is treated by one of the following:
A. Crotamiton B. Septran
C. Cetirizine D. Ampicillin

16. Molluscum contagiosum is mimicked by:
A. Herpes
B. Penicilliosis
C. Chromoblastomycoses
D. Sporotrichosis

17. The following is not used in treating warts:
A. Intralesional bleomycin
B. Podophyllin resin
C. 5% fluorouracil
D. Acyclovir

18. Nevirapine is a:
A. NRTI B. NNRTI
C. PI D. FI

19. The gold standard in diagnosis of genital herpes is based on:

A. Clinical features B. Tzanck smear
C. Monoclonal antibodies D. Viral culture

20. Which of the following is not true about acne therapy with isotretinoin?

A. Isotretinoin is the drug of choice
B. The dose is 1 mg/kg/d
C. The cumulative dose should be 120 mg/kg
D. The most common side effect is hair loss

21. The most diagnostic test for granuloma inguinale is:

A. Culture
B. Skin biopsy
C. Donovan bodies with safety pin appearance in tissue smear
D. Intradermal test

22. The following are characteristics of Treponema pallidum *except:*

A. Its length is 6 to 15 um
B. Its width is upto 0.25 um
C. It destroyed by drying
D. Can be easily cultured

23. Which is true about the treatment of bacillary angiomatosis true?

A. < CD 4 – 100
B. Erythromycin is given
C. Clofazemine is given
D. All are true

24. Which of the following is true about the treatment of scabies in pregnancy?

A. Ivermectin B. BHC
C. BB lotion D. Sulfur in calamine

25. Which of the following are specific dermatoses of HIV?

A. Exanthem of acute retroviral syndrome
B. PSO (Proximal Subungual Onychomycoses)
C. OHL (Oral Hairy Leucoplakia)
D. All of the above

26. A patient with psoriasis was started on systemic steroids. After stopping treatment, the patient developed generalized pustules all over the body. The causes of this can be all, *except:*

A. Iodide B. Steroids
C. Tar D. Salicylic acid

27. Satellite lesions are seen in which type of leprosy?

A. Tuberculoid leprosy
B. Lepromatous leprosy
C. Borderline tuberculoid leprosy
D. Histoid leprosy

28. All are features of dermatitis herpetiformis *except:*

A. Bilateral extensor distribution
B. Nikolsky sign positive
C. Papillary tip neutrophilic abscess
D. IgA granular pattern in dermis of affected area

29. All are true about Raynaud's diseases *except:*

A. Good prognosis
B. More in females
C. ANA test is positive
D. Raynaud's phenomenon is common presentation

30. Structure affected in scrofuloderma:

A. Bone B. Skin
C. Lymph node D. All of above

31. Which of the following is not true about lichen planus?

A. Excoriation B. Onychomadesis
C. Wickham's striae D. Itching

32. In an 8 days old child with no history of consanguinity in the parents, the mother reports blisters and peeling off of the skin at the site of handling and pressure. There was a similar history in the previous child which proved to be fatal. The diagnosis is:

A. Bullous pemphigoid
B. Congenital syphilis
C. Congenital epidermolysis bullosa
D. Letterer-Siwe disease

33. 30 years old Basanti presents with light brown lesions involving both her cheeks. This was associated with photosensitivity and oral erosions and arthritis, the most probable diagnosis:

A. SLE
B. Chloasma
C. Air-borne contact dermatitis
D. Photodermatitis

34. Babloo, 5 years, presents with small hypopigmented scaly macules on his cheek. *Some of his classmates also have similar lesions.* Which of the following is the most probable diagnosis?

A. Pityriasis alba
B. Pityriasis rosea
C. Pityriasis versicolor
D. Indeterminate leprosy

35. An 8 years old boy presents with a well-defined annular lesion over the buttock with central scarring that is gradually progressing over the last 8 months. He is a resident of Rajasthan. The diagnosis is:

A. Annular psoriasis
B. Leishmaniasis recidivans
C. Tinea corporis
D. Granuloma annulase

36. Imiquimod, an immunomodulator is useful in treatment of:

A. Herpes zoster
B. Condylomata acuminata
C. Psoriasis
D. Rheumatoid arthritis

37. Abnormal keratinisation of keratinocytes is called:

A. Dyskeratosis B. Parakeratosis
C. Hyperkeratosis D. Spongiosis

38. Dose of acyclovir in a patient suffering from herpes zoster is:

A. 200 mg, five times a day for 2 days
B. 400 mg, five times a day for 3 days
C. 600 mg, five times a day for 5 days
D. 800 mg, five times a day for 7 days

39. Hair perforation test is positive in infection with:

A. Trichophyton mentagrophytes
B. Microsporum canis
C. Epidermophyton floccosum
D. All of the above

40. Trichomycosis axillaris is caused by:

A. Trichophyton rubrum
B. Candida albicans
C. Parabacterium tenus
D. Corynebacterium minutissimum

41. Tuberculid is seen in:

A. Lupus vulgaris
B. Lichen scrofulosorum
C. Scrofuloderma
D. TBVC

42. Pityriasis rosea is a:

A. Chronic relapsing disease
B. Caused by dermatophyte
C. It is an autoimmune disease
D. Self resolving

43. Which of the following can be depressed:

A. Plaque B. Macule
C. Nodule D. Papule

44. Tyndall effect is present in:

A. Psoriasis
B. Lichen planus
C. Pemphigus
D. Dermatitis herpetiformis

45. A patient with antibodies to C-ANCA is suffering from involvement of kidney, liver, skin. The diagnosis is:

A PSS
B. SLE
C. RA
D. Wegener's granulomatosis

46. A young man aged 19 years develops multiple painless bleeding ulcers after sexual intercourse with a professional sex worker; likely diagnosis is:

A. Chancroid B. Herpes
C. Donovaniosis D. Traumatic ulcer

47. Which of the following conditions does not have pitting?

A. Psoriasis B. PRP
C. Trauma D. Lichen planus

48. A boy aged 8 years presents with a white, non-anesthetic, non scaly, hypopigmented macule on his face; likely diagnosis is:

A. Pityriasis alba
B. Pityriasis versicolor
C. Indeterminate leprosy
D. Pure neuritic leprosy

49. A 20 years old, male patient, from Jaipur, presents with an erythematous lesion on the cheek with central crusting; likely diagnosis is:

A. Baghdad boil
B. Lupus vulgaris
C. Chilblains
D. Leishmaniasis recidivans

50. A patient has bullous eruption on lower limb and trunk. Biopsy show subepidermal bullae. The correct statement is:

A. Pemphigoid
B. Pemphigus vulgaris
C. Impetigo
D. Rule out internal malignancy

51. All are true about herpes gestationis *except:*

A. Histologically similar to bullous pemphigoid
B. Usually occur in 2nd/3rd trimester
C. Confined to first pregnancy
D. Remits spontaneously

52. 'Pseudo chancre redux' is a clinical feature of:

A. Late syphilis
B. Early syphilis-chancre redux
C. Chancroid
D. Recurrent herpes simplex infection

Answers :

1. D	**2. C**	**3. D**	**4. B**
5. A	**6. C**	**7. D**	**8. A**
9. A	**10. A**	**11. D**	**12. C**
13. D	**14. C**	**15. B**	**16. B**
17. D	**18. B**	**19. D**	**20. D**
21. A	**22. D**	**23. D**	**24. D**
25. D	**26. C**	**27. C**	**28. B**
29. C	**30. D**	**31. A**	**32. C**
33. A	**34. C**	**35. B**	**36. B**
37. A	**38. D**	**39. A**	**40. D**
41. B	**42. D**	**43. A**	**44. B**
45. D	**46. C**	**47. D**	**48. C**
49. A	**50. D,A**	**51. C**	**52. A**

Explanatory Answers

TEST 1

(Only those questions are explained where the answers are a bit tedious to find in the text.)

1. The earliest test to be positive is FTA ABS in 2 weeks and VDRL is + 4 weeks after infection.
2. Itchy, grouped, extensor, IgA, granular > DH.
3. Pigmented macules can be seen in lichen planus, CALM of NF-1, but only in mastocytosis do they urticate, which is called Darier's sign.
4. AD-history of asthma, allergic rhinitis, itching OR allergy to food or family history of asthma.
5. Wood's lamp (-) are endothrix (TVS – tonsurans, violaceum and schoeinleinii), Scutula are seen in favus – caused by the schoeinleinii species.
6. It is seen in groin, flexures and is caused by corynebacterium (coral red fluorescence).
7. Non scaly macules is leprosy and the most common cause in India is indeterminate leprosy.
8. The earliest is subungual hyperkeratosis but the most classical is oil drop sign.
9. This is seen in S corneum but the collection of neutrophils in S granulosum (Kogoj pustule) is MORE SPECIFIC.
16. The most common cause of allergic contact dermatitis in the world– Ni/Co, most common in India housewives is detergent, in farmers it is parthenium.
17. Cause of scarring alopecia –DLE, lichen planus, trauma, favus and pseudopelade.
18. Black hairy tongue caused because of broad spectrum antibiotics.
23. To monitor therapy in leprosy the tool used is MI (becomes 0 in 6 weeks) in syphilis it is VDRL.
33. You have to treat the clothes, lindane or permethrin can be used in CONJUNCTION but this choice can be given also if it is an MCQ in PGI exam.
35. **Pregnancy**, 3rd trimester, **in primi**, can recur, heals spontaneously, C3 is seen (Herpes gestationis).
39. It is caused by Parvovirus.
40. If it is PGI exam both DLE and LP is the answer.
42. Bullous pyoderma gangrenosum is a vasculitis seen in malignancy, here it is just a pyoderma.
43. Again if this is a question of PGI all except peripheral neuritis, the others are rare causes of lagophthalmos.
44. Again if it is PGI a rare cause is P vulgaris.
47. The ideal choice in male is 5% minoxidil + finasteride 1 mg. In females it is 2% minoxidil.
51. All infectious organisms can be cultured except syphilis leprosy.
52. Most common skin lesion is CALM, most common benign skin tumor neurofibroma, most common CNS tumor is optic glioma. Most specific skin lesion is lisch nodules.
56. T facei is the diagnosis.
57. A rare indication of Wood's lamp in a fair individual with vitiligo.
62. This and amorolofine nail lacquer is used for nail fungus.
65. Immediate pigment darkening on exposure to sunlight is because of UV A. This normally disappears in 30 min.
66. Endothrix – corresponds to a clinical appearance of Black Dot – Trichophytum sp.
78. Itchy, tense, bulla, IgG – Bullous pemhigoid.
81. Plaque, annular in shape, with crusting and indurations at:
    - *Lupus vulgaris* plaque, annular in shape, with crusting and indurations at the periphery and scarring at the center.
    - +Rajasthan-Leishmaniasis recidivans plaque
    - Annular in shape, with itching –Tinea corporis plaque
    - Annular in shape, with sensory loss –Leprosy.
83. Multiple hypo anesthetic mildly erythematous large plaques with elevated margins, ulnar and lateral popliteal nerves on both sides were enlarged—BT, multiple hypo-anesthetic macules, ulnar and lateral popliteal nerves on enlarged—BL.
86. IgG – reticular and suprabasal basal layer—P vulgaris.
    IgG— Upper epidermis—Foliaceous.
    IgG—Linear only BMZ—Bullous Pemphigoid.
    C3—Herpes gestationis.
    Ig A—linear – chronic bullous dermatoses of childhood.
    Ig A—granular – Dermatitis Herpetiformis.
87. (i) Erythema and swelling of the periorbital region-HELIOTROPE SIGN.
    (ii) Papules and plaques on the dorsolateral aspect of forearms and knuckles gottrons sign.
    (iii) There was no muscle weakness—AMYOPATHIC VARIANT.
89. Sexually active male – Secondary syphilis as a P rosea like rash can be seen in syphilis also.

TEST 2

1. It is a diagnostic test ONLY IN RIDLEY JOPLING classification.
4. It is bulla below the epidermis.
12. Diarrhoea, in a diabetic alcoholic, with photosensitivity, casal necklace and glove and gauntlet sign seen in pellagra.
15. This option is correct only for cong. syphilis.
18. TPHA test as IgG ab which crosses the fetoplacental barrier and thus the child is falsely positive (TPHA).

IgM FTAABS is the best serological marker as IgM does not cross the barrier and indicates actue infection.

20. The earlist is thinning of nail plate, f/b longitudinal pigmentation, pup tent sign, onychoschizia and then loss of nail *onychomadesis*.
22. If patient is married – Azithromycin as it is safe even if the patient gets pregnant accidentally.
25. Trichomoniasis is characterized by polymorphs.
31. Inhibits the 5 alpha reductase type 2 receptor.
32. Pautriers microabscess are common – composed of lymphocyte.
    It has an indolent course and good prognosis—The latter is wrong (good prognosis).
    . It presents with diffuse erythroderma; Sezary syndrome.
33. GVH acute: Skin, liver, GIT.
    Chronic: Lichenoid scleroderma like.
34. Ingestion of protein (sea food, nuts) dyspnoea (mucosal swelling).
52. Child presented with overnight rash all over body. 2 weeks ago he had an episode of abdominal *pain*. There was *mild pallor* and *no hepatosplenomegaly.* What is the likely diagnosis.
    The most common cause of non drug induced infectious rash in children is enteroviral and its features are either URTI or diarrhoea.
53. Child presented with *petechial* rash all over body with ecchymosis on the lower limb. 2 weeks ago he had an episode of *abdominal pain.* There was *severe pallor*, weakness and *no hepatosplenomegaly.* What is the likely diagnosis?
    Aplastic anemia.
54. Child presented with petechial rash all over body. 2 weeks ago he had an episode of *abdominal pain*. There was *mild pallor*, weakness and *no hepatosplenomegaly*. What is the likely diagnosis?

    ITP

    (The answer to this question actually depends on the signs mentioned) ecchymoses is seen more commonly in plastic anemia.
    - ITP—purpura.
    - Aplastic anemia—Severe pallor, weakness, abdominal pain.
    - Enteroviral rash—Causes urt or abdominal symptoms.
    - Inf mononucleosis—Rash, most common drug ampicillin, ¼ have petechiae on plate, fever, malaise, LN spleen.
    - Drug—Within 1-3 weeks, itch, eosinophilia, serum sickness.
    - Kawasaki—Fever, rash extremity, rash trunk, conjunctivitis, oral strawberry tongue, LN, heart.

TEST 3

1. Exposed sites, child, more in rainy season – insect bite reaction-papular urticaria.
11. This is because according to syndromic approach both chlamydia and gonorrhoea cause the disease and 2 gm covers both organisms.
13. To distinguish BP from EB acquisita.
15. The louse has commensal bacteria in its gut that produce vitamin on which the louse survives, when the louse ingests blood with septran the commensal in its gut die due to which the louse dies.
20. *The most common side effect is cheilitis and dry skin.*
24. The safest agent in pregnancy and infants is sulfur f/b permethrin.
34. • Hypopigmented scaly macules on his cheek—P alba.
    - Hypopigmented non-scaly macules on his cheek—Leprosy.
    - *Some of his classmates also have similar lesions*–indicates an infectious etiology and face involvement is seen in P versicolor in children.
38. 200 mg, five times a day for 2 days—Herpes genitalis.

Part VII

Selected Pages from *Comprehensive Textbook of Dermatology*
(Written for 'CET' 2012)

The **process of cornification involves** (1) synthesis of *lamellar granules* and distinctive *proteins*, e.g., differentiation-specific keratins, filaggrin, loricrin, involucrin, and desmosomal proteins that are cross-linked by transglutaminases, and (2) changes progressively of nuclei, cytoplasmic organelles, plasma membranes, and desmosomes.

Basal Layer

The **basal row** of keratinocytes consists of cuboidal or low columnar cells that contains larger oval nuclei and more basophilic cytoplasm than the more mature keratinocytes above them.

- This deepest layer of the epidermis is made up of a single layer of columnar cells which have a basophilic cytoplasm and an oval nucleus.
- These cells are firmly attached to the *lamina densa* of the basement membrane with the help of *hemidesmosomes.*
- The distribution of keratins (K) in the various layers of epidermis is as follows:
  Basal cell layer—K5/K14
  Spinous—K1/K10, K5/K14
  Granular—K2/K11

MCQ

- The basal cells contain melanin – the amount of melanin present in the basal cells is reflected as the skin colour.
- In the light skinned the melanin granules, *melanosomes* are barely visible while in the dark skinned there are innumerable distinct granules predominantly forming supra nuclear caps.

Spinous or Prickle Layer

- This layer, which lies above the basal layer, is made up of polygonal cells forming a mosaic of 5-10 layers; they are attached to each other by interlocking cytoplasmic processes, numerous *desmosomes* (attachment plaques) and the *intercellular cement* (of glycoproteins).
- It is the presence of desmosomes which gives the cells of this layer an appearance of prickles (under the light microscope).
- Under the electron – microscope, these cells are filled with *tonofilaments.*
- The cells of the upper part of this layer are filled with *odland* or *lamellar bodies.*

Granular Layer

- The granular layer is made up of 1-3 layers.
- The cytoplasm of granular cells is filled with *tonofilaments* and basophilic *keratohyaline* granules – these two structures gradually merge during keratinisation.
- The lysosomal enzymes of the granular cells destroy the cell nuclei and intracytoplasmic organelles, as the granular layer cells become horny cells.

The spinous zone merges with horizontally oriented diamond-shaped cells filled with coarse, basophilic keratohyaline granules, i.e., cells of the granular zone. Keratohyaline granules are made up of profilaggrin, an electron-dense protein, loricrin, and keratin intermediate filaments.

Near the top of the spinous zone, **lamellar granules** (also referred to as Odland bodies) appear near the Golgi apparatus, navigate the cytoplasm, and fuse with the plasma membrane, where their contents are discharged from keratinocytes into intercellular spaces. These granules contain free sterols, polar lipids, e.g., phospholipids and glucosylceramides (the precursors of ceramides), and several hydrolytic enzymes, e.g., lipases, glycosidases, and acid phosphatase. After contents of lamellar granules are released into intercellular spaces, they are restructured into lamellae that provide the basic structure for an effective epidermal barrier to permeability.

Desmosomes (Fig. 1.6)

Desmosomes consist of a number of proteins, among them being desmoglein 1 and 3, desmoplakin, plakoglobin and desmosomal cadherins. When the function of desmosomes is impaired, keratinocytes tend to become detached from one another and, in the process, assume a *round shape*.

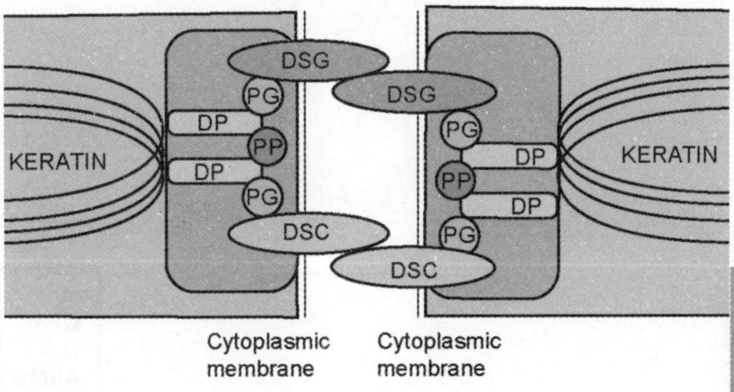

Fig. 1.6: Desmosome

DP=Desmoplakin
PG=Plakoglobin
PP=Periplakin
DSG= Desmoglein
DSC=Desmocollin

The phenomenon occurs in conditions as disparate as **pemphigus vulgaris** (autoantibodies against desmoglein 3), **pemphigus foliaceus** (autoantibodies against desmoglein 1), and **staphylococcal scalded skin syndrome** in which exfoliatins produced by the Gram-positive cocci compromise desmosomes severely.

MCQ

SECTION - 1

3

size. It is then triggered to enter the *S Phase* or the phase of DNA synthesis. The cell next enters the G_2 or *post-synthetic phase* and finally divides in the *M phase*. One of the daughter cells moves up to become a keratinocyte, while the other enters the G_1 *phase* (sometimes the G_0 or *resting stage*). Various factors control the epidermal cell proliferation (*epidermopoiesis*). Cytokines, growth factors and hormones influence the rate of epidermopoiesis.

- Normal *cell cycle time 311 hours (60-450 hours).*
- Time required for basal cell to reach stratum corneum—*53 days.*
- Time required for cell to be shed off from stratum corneum—*14 days.*
- Total cell proliferation time–52-75 days.* ← MCQ

- They may also insert into amorphous bodies in superficial dermis known as ANCHORING PLAQUES, or more typically curve back to have a second insertion in LAMINA DENSA.
- They vary widely in individuals and vary in density in different regions of body.
- The antigenic components of lamina fibroreticularis are:
  - EBA Ag (in Type VII collagen).
  - 285 kDa protein (some cases of LINEAR IgA BULLOUS DERMATOSIS).

Table 1.1: Basement membrane antigens

Constituents	*Location*	*Genodermatosis*	*Autoimmune bullous disease*
Keratins 5 and 14	Basal keratinocyte	EB simplex	None
$\alpha_6\beta_4$ integrin	DEJ	JEB-pyloric atresia	None
BP180	DEJ	GABEB	BP, CP, HG, LPP
Plectin	Hemidesmosome	EBS-MD	BP
BP230 (→ MCQ AIIMS PGI)	Hemidesmosome		BP
Laminin 5	Lamina lucida	Junctional EB	CP
Type VII collagen	Sublamina densa	Dystrophic EB	EBA, BSLE, LAD

BP—Bullous Pemphigoid
CP—Cicatrical Pemphigoid
HG—Herpes Gestationis
LPP—Lichen Planus Pemphigoides
EBA—Epidermolysis Bullosa Acquisita
BSLE—Bullous SLE
LAD—Linear IgA Dermatosis

Table 1.2: Autoimmune bullous diseases—Target antigens

Disease	*Target Ag (M wt in kDa)*	*Site of Ag*
P.foliaceous	Desmoglein 1 (160)	Desmosomes of upper epidermis
IgA Pemphigus (→ MCQ AIIMS PGI)	Desmocollin 1	Desmosomes (transmembrane)
P.vulgaris	Desmoglein 3 (130)	Desmosomes of lower epidermis
EBA	Type VII collagen (290)	Anchoring fibrils
Paraneoplastic pemphigus	Desmoplakin 1 (250)	Cytoplasmic plaques
Bullous pemphigoid	BPAg1(230) BPAg2 (180)	Hemidesmosome transmembrane protein
Pemphigoid gestationis	BPAg2 (180)	
DH	Transglutaminase 2	Unknown structure most likely keratin
Linear IgA disease	LAD -1 ladinin (97) 285 kDa	Anchoring filament Sublamina densa
Ocular CP	Not named	Conjunctiva
Cicatricial pemphigoid	BPAg2 (180) Epiligrin	Against 3 subunit of laminin 5
—	—	—

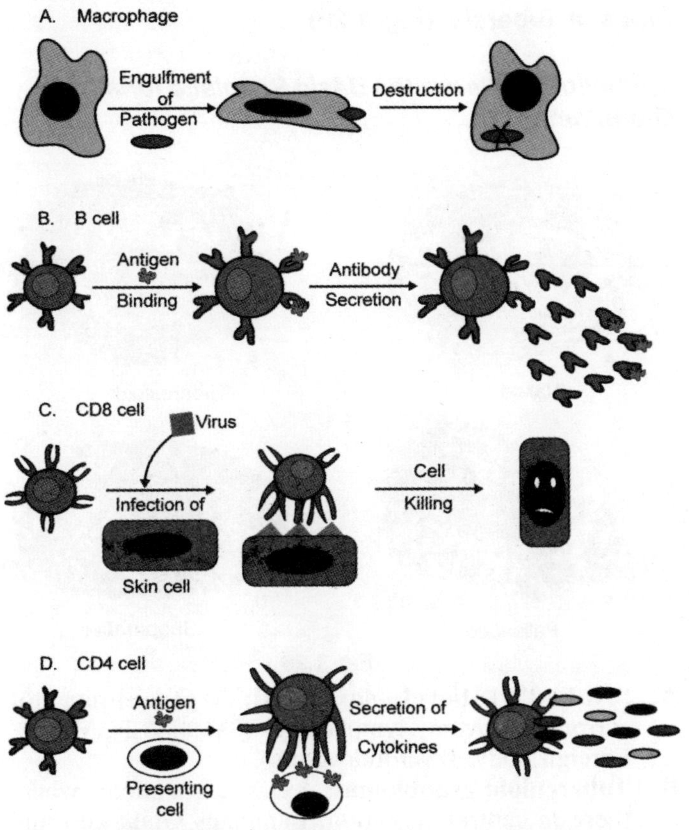

Figs. 1.23A to 1.23D: Immune cell response

(called "self antigens"). It is now clear that CD_4 T cells are also a main target for the human immunodeficiency virus (HIV) that causes AIDS. Understanding how to control CD_4 T cells will allow us to develop better vaccines, abolish many forms of autoimmunity, and control allergies.

REFERENCES

- L.P. Gartner and J.L. Hiatt: Color Textbook of Histology, 3rd edn., Elsevier, 2007, p 331-336.
- Junqueria and Carneiro: Basic Histology Text and Atlas, 11th edn., McGraw-Hill, 2005, p 361.
- Histologic Diagnosis of Inflammatory Skin Diseases. An Algorithmic Method Based on Pattern Analysis, 3rd edn. *A. Bernard Ackerman, MD, Almut Böer, MD, Bruce Bennin, MD and Geoffrey J. Gottlieb, MD* 2005.
- Rook's Textbook of Dermatology; D. A. Burns , S. M. Breathnach, Neil Cox, Christopher E, Griffith's 7th edn 2004.
- Fitzpatrick's Dermatology in General Medicine, 6th edn 2003.
- Lever's Histopathology of the Skin by David E Elder, Rosalie Elenitsas, Bernett L Johnson, George F Murphy, 9th edn. 2004.
- Thieme's Pocket Dermatology 2006 by Wolfram Sterry, Walter Burgdorf, Ralf Paus.
- Veedon Textbook of Histopathology.
- Ackerman Textbook of Histopathology.
- Morschella Textbook of Dermatology.

Essentials of Histopathology

DEFINITIONS OF HISTOLOGICAL TERMS

1. Abscess

Definition:
- Neutrophils are joined by products of necrosis and degeneration.

Example:
- Munro's microabscess and spongiform pustule of Kogoj-Psoriasis.

2. Acantholysis

A process whereby epithelial cells, as a consequence of loss of connections (desmosomes) between them, separate from one another.

Cause

- Immunoglobulins.
- Neutrophils on keratocytes in the lower part of the epidermis.
- Vesicants.

Primary

- Pemphigus vulgaris.
- Hailey Hailey disease.
- Squamous cell carcinoma.
- Warty dyskeratoma (acantholytic dyskeratotic acanthoma).
- Epidermal nevus typified by foci of acantholytic dyskeratosis.
- Darier's disease.

Secondary

- Dermatitis herpetiformis.
- Linear IgA dermatosis.
- Bullous lupus erythematosus.
- Impetigo.
- Majocchi's "granuloma".
- Herpes.

3. Acanthosis

- Increase in number of spinous cells—psoriasis.
- Size of spinous cells—lichen planus.
- Number and size of spinous cells—lichen simplex chronicus.

4. Dyskeratosis (Fig. 1.24)

- Dyskeratotic cells have pyknotic nuclei and eosinophilic cytoplasm.
- Filaments of keratin in perinuclear aggregation.

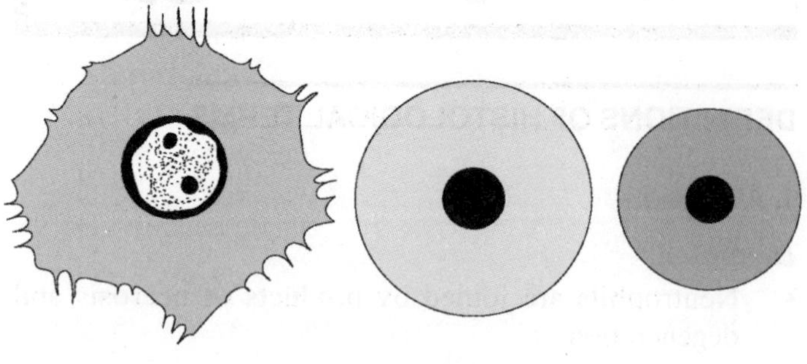

Fig. 1.24: Progression from (Normal) keratinocyte to dyskeratosis

- Grover's disease.
- Verrucous stage of Incontinentia pigmenti.
- Neoplastic diseases–Bowen's disease and subungual keratoacanthoma.
- Genodermatoses–Darier's disease.
- Cystic conditions such as warty dyskeratoma.

5. Granuloma (Fig. 1.25)

A collection of histiocytes, usually epithelioid ones:

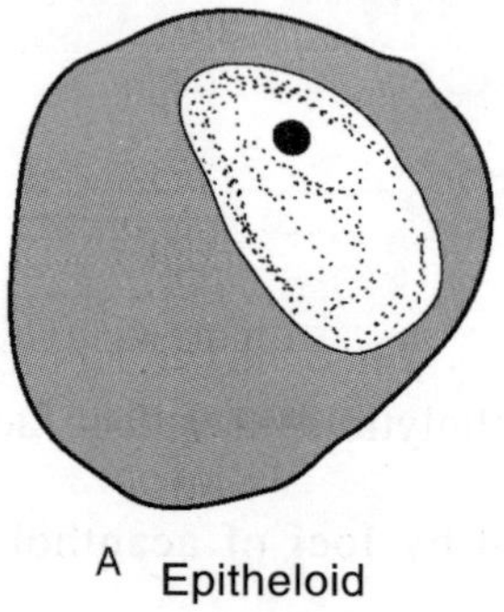

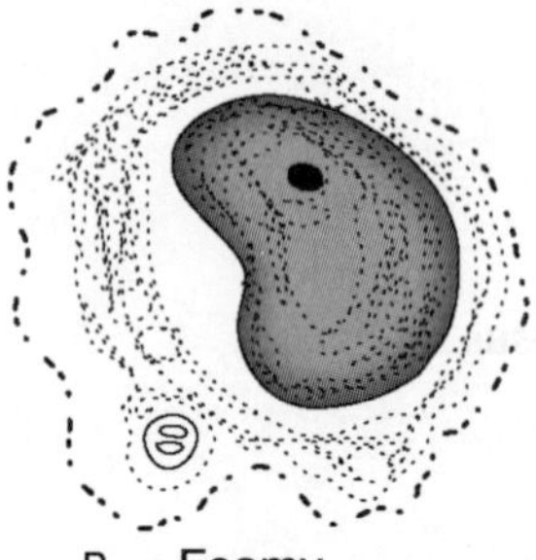

Figs. 1.25A and 1.25B

- Epithelioid histiocytes–TT/BT (Fig 1.25A).
- Foamy histiocytes–Lepromatous leprosy, xanthogranulomas (Fig. 1.25B).
- Multinucleate histiocytes (Langhans', Touton and foreign body).

Types of Tubercle (Fig. 1.26)

Epithelioid Cells are the Basic Requisite for all Granuloma

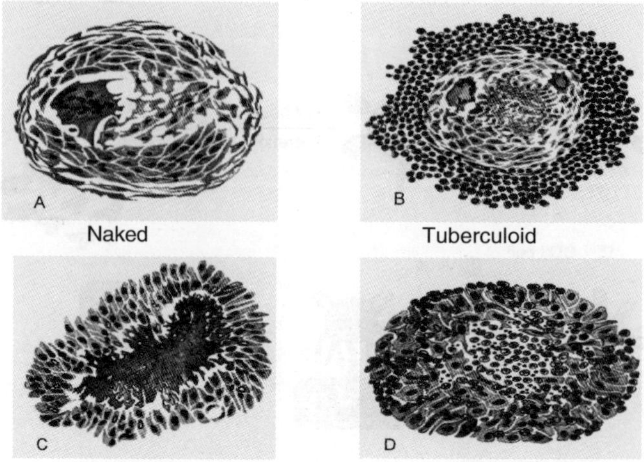

Fig. 1.26

A. **"Naked" tubercle-sarcoidal:** A granuloma not surrounded by any lymphocytes (Sarcoidosis, MRSA, Foreign body, L scrofulosorum).
B. **Tuberculoid granulomas:** A classic granuloma where there is central caseation, Langhans Giant cell and surrounded by Lymphocytes (TB, LMDF, Cryptococcosis, Histoplasmosis).
C. **Palisaded:** A granuloma composed of alternating bands on mucin, collagen and epithelioid cells (interstitial Garnuloma annulare).
D. **Suppurative:** A granuloma composed of neutrophils.

6. Hypergranulosis

- *Increased thickness of the granular zone of an epidermis.*

Examples:

- Lichen planus.
- Lichen simplex chronicus.
- Bullous congenital ichthyosiform erythroderma.

7. Hyperkeratosis

- Increase in the layers of stratum corneum – seen in psoriasis and other psoriasiform disorders.

Basket-Weave Orthokeratosis (Fig. 1.27)

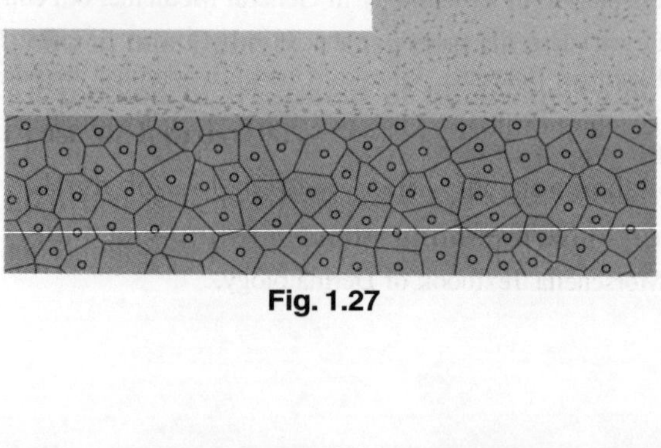

Fig. 1.27

10. Superficial Perivascular Dermatitis Important Patterns (Figs. 1.31-1.33)

Sup Perivascular Psoriasiform

- Lymphocytes–Chronic Atopic Dermatitis.
- Plasma cells–Secondary Syphilis.
- Eosinophil–Chronic ACD.
- Neutrophil– Psoriasis Vulgaris.

Sup Perivascular-Lichenoid

- Lymphocytes–Lichen planus.
  Lymphocytes *plus*.
  i. Plasma cells–Secondary syphilis.

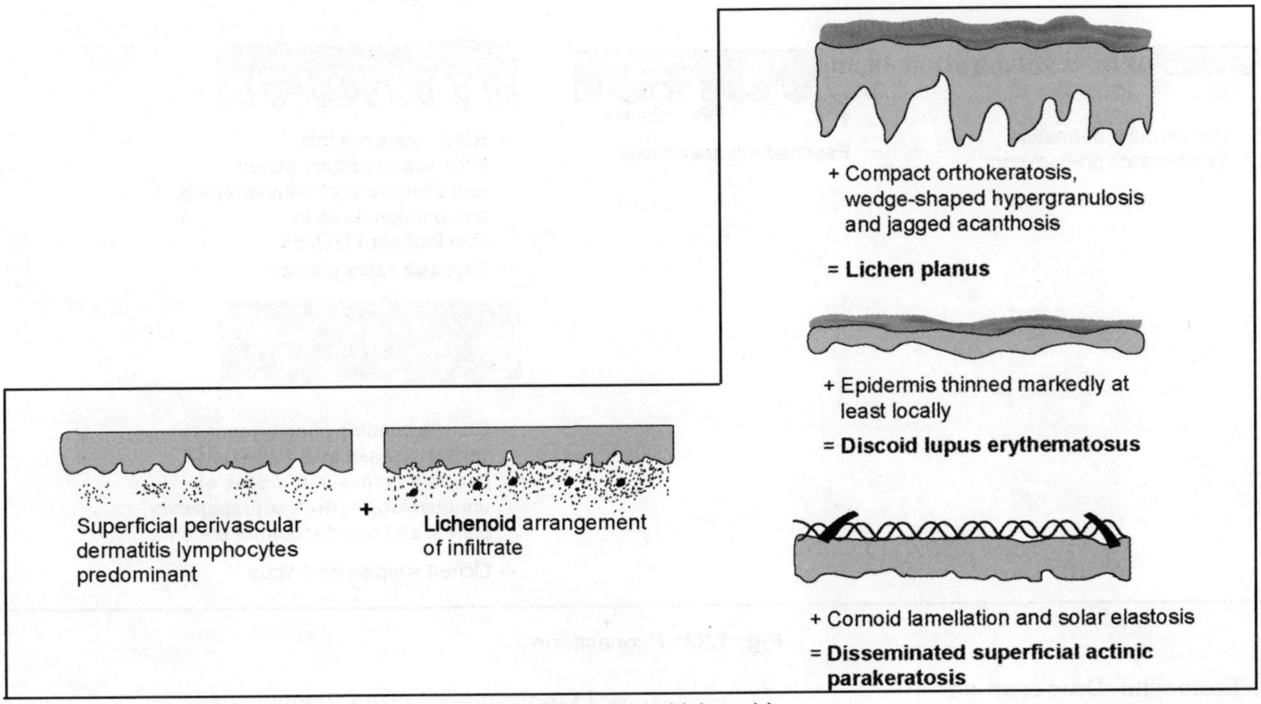

Fig. 1.31: Lichenoid

MCQs asked in All Exam

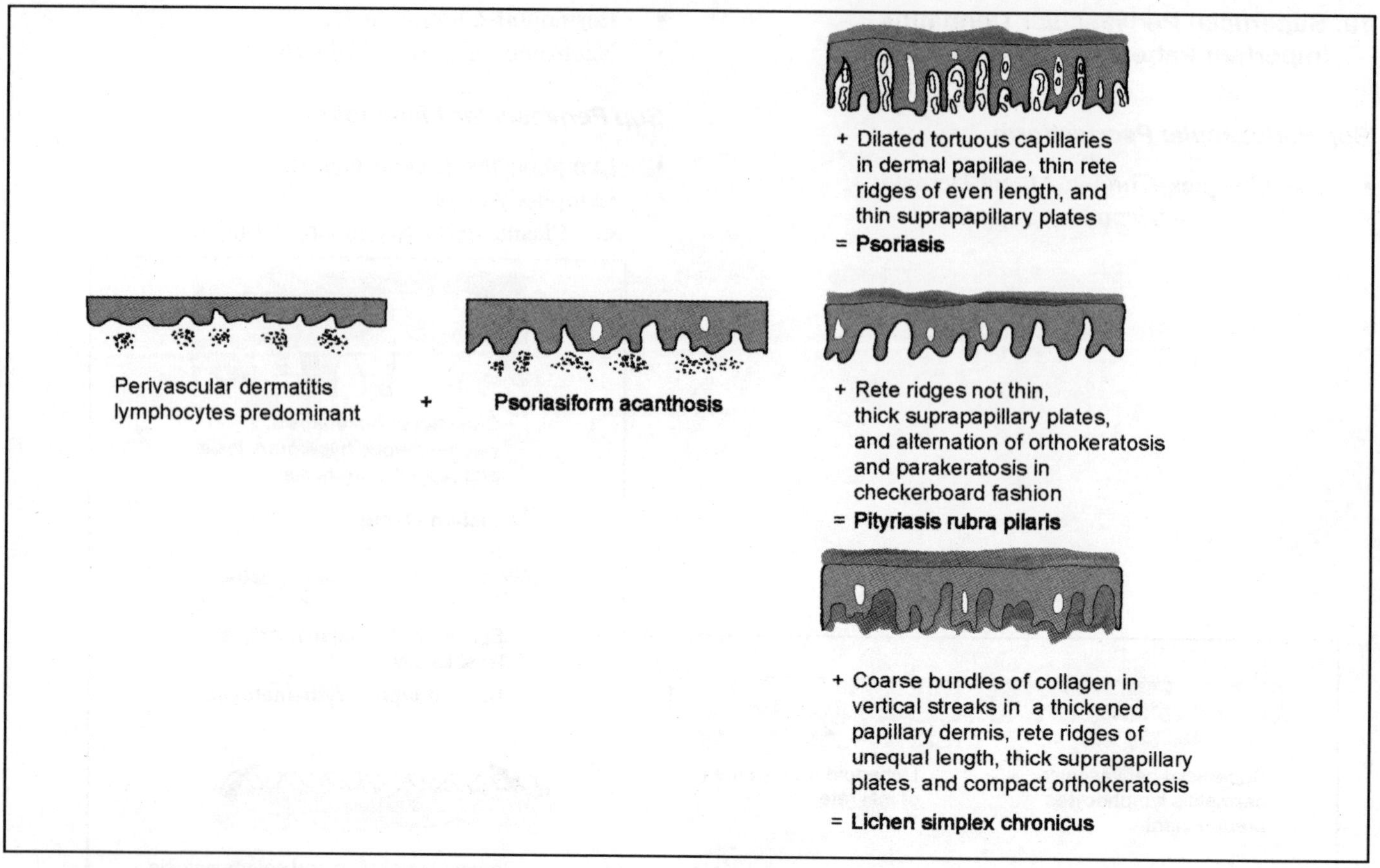

Fig. 1.33: Psoriasiform

ii. Eosinophil–Drug eruption.
iii. Melanocyte–Post inflammatory hyperpigmentation.
iv. Histiocytes–L nitidus.
v. Mast cells–Urticaria pigmentosa.

11. Interface Dermatitis

- **"Vacuolar"** (a sprinkling of inflammatory cells, usually lymphocytes, in conjunction with vacuolar alteration along that interface).
- **"Lichenoid"** (a bandlike infiltrate of inflammatory cells, usually lymphocytes, that, in association with vacuolar alteration, tends to obscure the interface).

Examples:

- Apoptic cells–Erythema multiforme.
- Minimal apotopsis–Dermatomyosistis.
- Variable–drug eruption.
- BMZ thickening–LE.

12. Vesicular Dermatitis

MCQs asked in All Exam

a. *The level of split*

i. Intraepidermal (Fig. 1.34)
ii. Subepidermal (Fig. 1.35)
Scant Cells=Porphyria Cutanea Tarda
Lymphocyte= Lichen Planus
Eosinophil = Bullous Pemphigoid
Neutrophil = Dermatitis Herpetiformis
Mast cell = Urticaria Pigmentosa

iii. Intra- and Subepidermal (Fig. 1.36)

Methenamine silver

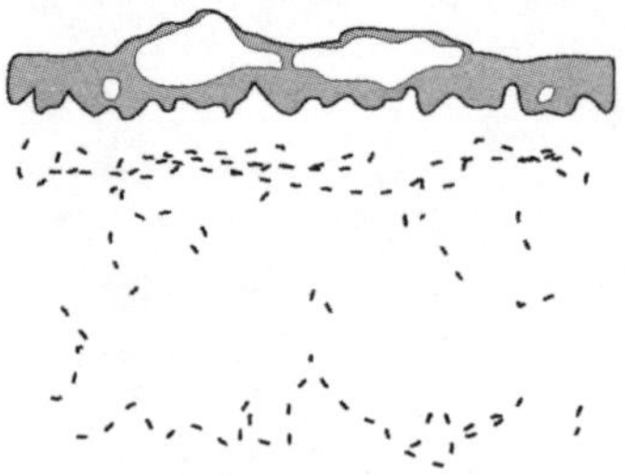

Fig. 1.34: Intraepidermal

Fungi, basement membrane

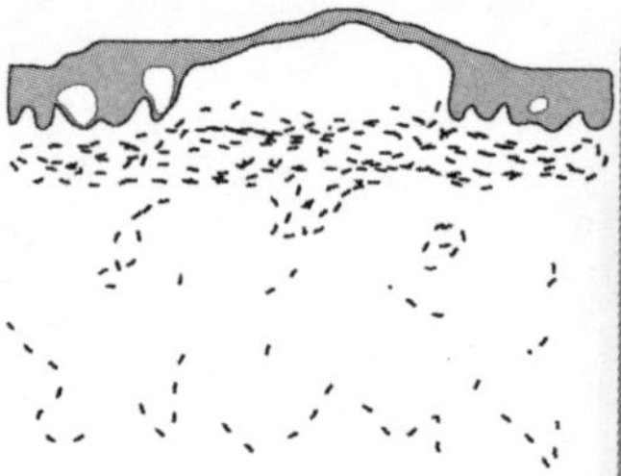

Fig. 1.35: Subepidermal

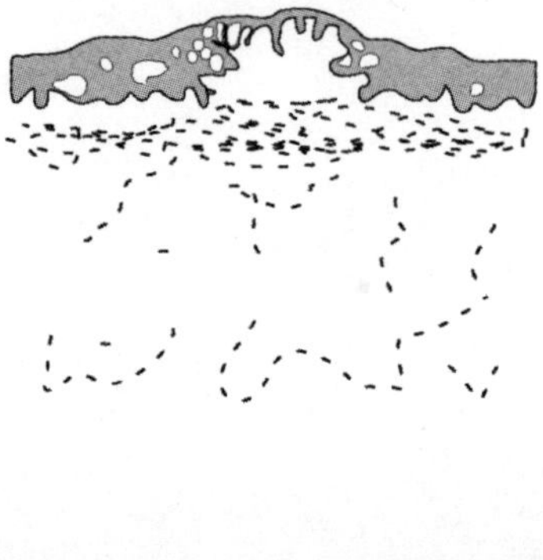

Fig. 1.36: Intra and Subepidermal

2. Endothrix—Hyphae are inside the hair shaft (Fig. 2.37). Wood's light negative.
3. Favus—Special variant.

Species

- **Ectothrix–***T mentagrophytes, M canis, T verrucosum.*
- **Endothrix–***T tonsurans, T violaceum.*
- **Favus–T schoenleinii.**
- Most common type in USA—*T tonsurans.*
- Most common type in India—*T violaceum.*

MCQ asked in all exam

Clinical types:

- **Non-inflammatory**, human or epidemic type **(grey patch)** *T mentagrophytes, M audouinii.*
- **Inflammatory** type (Kerion)—*M canis.*
- **'Black dot'**—*T tonsurans.*
- **Favus.**
- **Rare (Agminate** folliculitis).

1. Non-inflammatory, human or epidemic type (grey patch) (Fig. 2.38).
   The clinical picture is of an area of hair loss, with itching with a grayish hue because of the external coating of the hair shafts by spores and hyphae.
2. Non-inflammatory (Alopecia areata type).
3. Inflammatory type (Kerion)—*M canis* (Fig. 2.39). This is characterized by a painful nodule on the scalp with hair loss usually caused by zoophilic species.
4. Favus—This variant is seen in Jammu and Kashmir and is characterized by scutulae, a yellowish crust at the base of the hair, scarring alopecia (Fig. 2.40) and on KOH, air spaces in a linear fashion are seen in the hair shaft.

Treatment

- Oral antifungal agents are necessary because topical agents are not able to penetrate deeply enough into the hair follicle; griseofulvin is the first choice.
- Oral terbinafine and itraconazole are good alternatives (although more expensive).

Treatment

- Griseofulvin 10-15 mg/kg/d × 6-8 weeks.
- Terbinafine 5 mg/kg/d × 2-4 weeks.
- **Itraconazole**
  Continuous 5 mg/kg/d × 2-4 weeks.
  Pulse 5 mg/kg/d for 1 week/month × 1-3 pulses.
- **Fluconazole**
  Continuous 6 mg/kg/d × 20 days.
  Pulse 6 mg/kg/dose once per week × 8-12 weeks.
- Adjunct. therapy with antifungal shampoos.

T. CORPORIS

- Infection of non-hairy skin.
- Most common causative agents:
  - *T. rubrum.*
  - *M. canis.*
  - *T. mentagrophytes.*

Clinical Types

- **Classical annular:** Peripheral scaling and central clearing (Fig. 2.41).
- **Inflammatory:** *Trichophyton verrucosum* infection, usually from cattle, produces severe inflammatory response with uniformly round, raised lesions with moist and pustular surface, follicular pustules within hair follicles, possible secondary bacterial infection, brown hyperpigmentation, and scarring. *Trichophyton rubrum* infection produces Majocchi's granuloma, follicular papulopustules or inflammatory nodules, granulomatous nodules with necrotic areas, unusual hyphal forms, and mucinous coating.

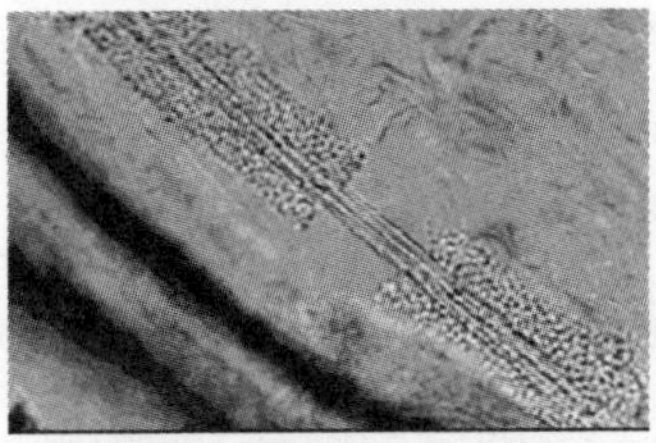

Fig. 2.36: Spores lying outside the hair shaft—ectothrix

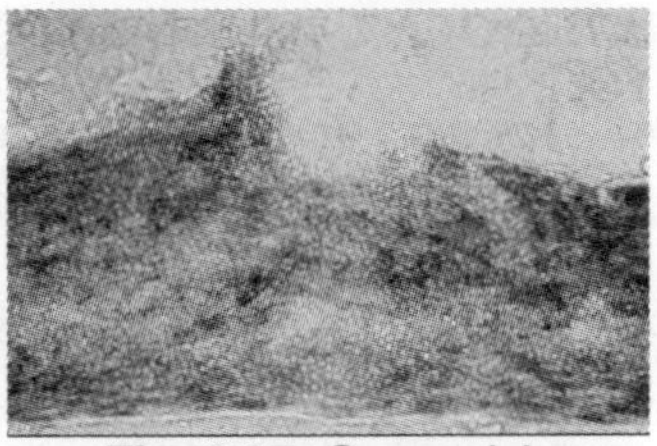

Fig. 2.37: Spores lying inside the hair shaft—endothrix

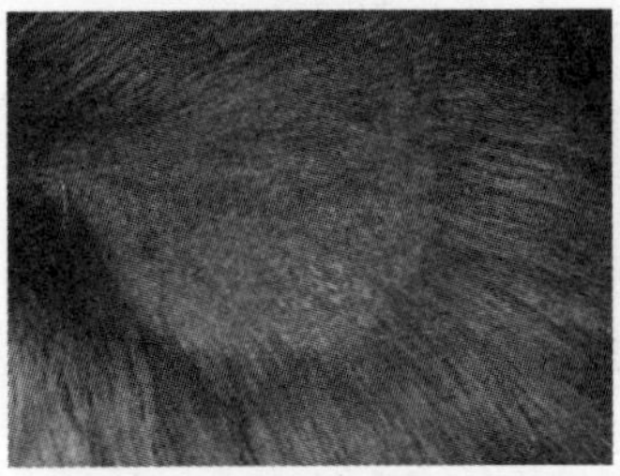

Fig. 2.38: Greyish area of alopecia–due to the coating of spores of the hair shaft (Grey patch)

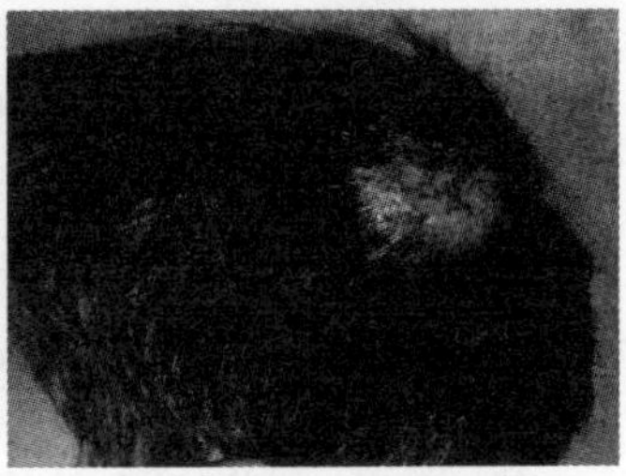

Fig. 2.39: Painful inflammatory nodule (Kerion)

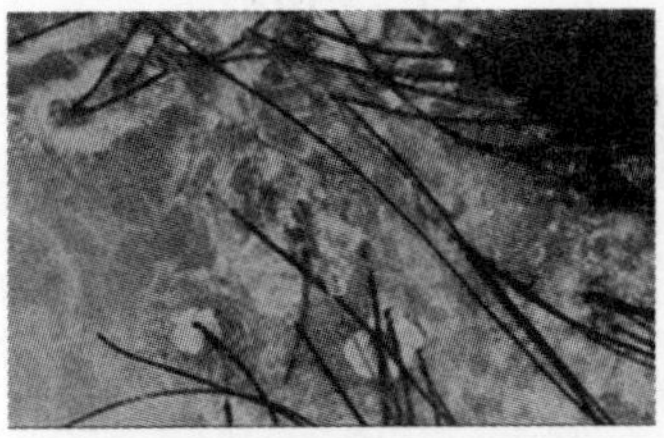

Fig. 2.40: Yellowish crust engulfing multiple hair (Favus)

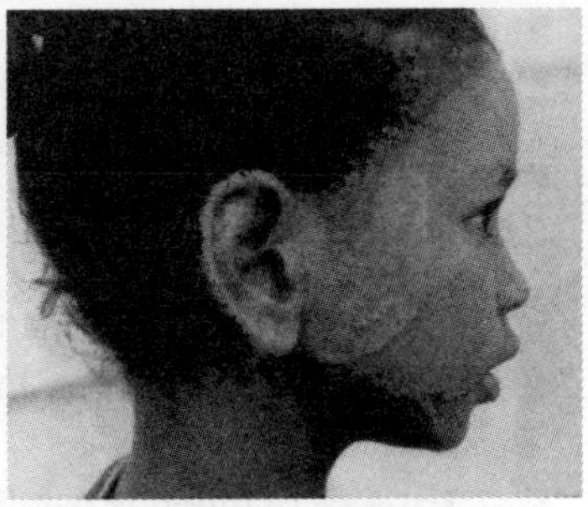

Fig. 2.41: Peripheral spread and central clearing (Tinea corporis)

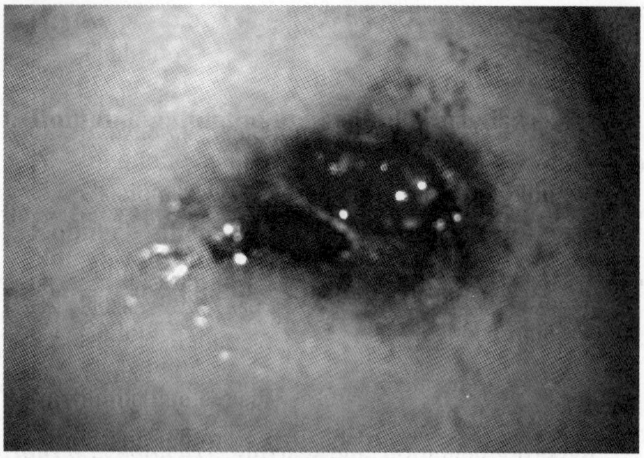

Fig. 2.71: Nontender abscesses perforate the skin, forming ulcers

IATROGENIC IMMUNIZATION TUBERCULOSIS

- Primary inoculation complex, scrofuloderma, lupus vulgaris, exfoliative dermatitis or acute miliary tuberculosis.
- Exfoliative dermatitis after B.C.G. vaccination (in immunodeficient patients).

TUBERCULOUS MASTITIS

- Rare form of tuberculosis involving the breast.
- Present with a nontender, cold abscess.

TUBERCULIDS

- Symmetrical, generalized **exanthem** in the skin of a tuberculous patient.
- Due to an **allergic or hypersensitivity reaction** to the tubercle bacillus or one of its constituent parts.

Tuberculids are:

- Lichen scrofulosrum.
- Papulonecrotic tuberculid.
- Erythema induratum.

Very Imp common MCQ

Criterion

- Positive tuberculin skin test.
- Tuberculous involvement of lymph nodes or internal viscera or both.
- Absence of tubercle bacilli from skin biopsy and culture.
- Skin lesions that heal on remission of the tuberculous infection.

Table 2.8: Clinical findings under Ridley Jopling types

Classification according to Ridley Jopling scheme

	TT	*BT*	*BB*	*BL*	*LL*
Cutaneous lesion	Hypopig/erythematous macules/ plaques **well defined**, **regular-border** dry scaly **saucer right way up** Complete loss of hair/sweat **Anaesthetic.** **Number usually < 3** Nerve to patch Nerve Abscess	Hypopig/erythematous macules/ plaques **well-ill** defined, **irregular** margins, **satellite lesions.** Impaired/complete loss of sweating/hair **Hypoaesthesia** .<10 Numerous Nerves Assymetrical Nerve Abscess	Morphology of tuberculoid as well as lepromatous **Swiss cheese** **Punched out** **Geographic** Parial loss of sweat hair Hypo-normoaethesia Numerous B/L sym Countable Numerous Nerves asymmetrical	Variable morphology with papules Shiny to dry **Inverted Saucer** margin well defined Partial to no loss hair and sweat Hypo-normoaethesia Numerous B/L sym Uncountable Symmetrical	Infiltration, madarosis leonine facies, hypopig/erythematous macules, plaque papules nodules. Margins ill defined No loss of sweat/hair Normoaesthesia Numerous B/L sym - Uncountable Symmetrical
Immunology (lepromin)	Strongly positive (+++)	Weakly positive (+ or ++)	**Negative** (–)	Negative (–)	Negative (–)
Histopath	**Compact granuloma** (tuberculoid) hugging or eroding epidermis. **Cutaneous nerves → destroyed** Langhan Giant Cell	Tuberculoid granuloma less compact than TT. Subepid, **grenz-zone appears.** Nerves → cellular infiltrate	Diffuse epitheloid cell granuloma Grenz zone + nerves → infiltrated epitheloid cell Langhans (-)	Granuloma composed of macrophages + lymphocytes. Grenz zone + Nerves **onion peeling nerve**	Thinned epider. Diffuse lepromatous foamy macrophages few. Lymphocytes + plasma cells. Grenz zone cut nerves are preserved **Virchow cell**
Epilhelioid cells	1+	1 +	1+		
Lymphocytes	3+	2+	1+	3+	0-1+
Langhans' cells	3+	2+	—	—	—
Touton giant cells	—	—	—	—	1+
Globi					1+
Foam cells				1+	2+
CD_4+/CD_8+	1.35 1	—	—	—	0.48 0.50
M. leprae	1+ (60%+)	2+	2+ 3+	3+	4+ (95%+)
PGL-1 antibodies					
AFB(BI)	0-1+	2-3+	4-5 +	4-6+	globi/normal skin

SALIENT CLINICAL FEATURES OF RIDLEY JOPLING TYPES

1. Tuberculoid (TT)

Single or few, asymmetrical, well-defined, hypopigmented, erythematous or copper-coloured patches.

Clinical

1. The **entire patch (Fig. 2.75) only its edge is raised (Fig. 2.76)** above the surrounding skin.
2. **Hypopigmented patches** not raised above the level of the surrounding skin.
3. Psoriasiform rarely.

Clinical Features

- Lice 1-2 mm appear as brownish-grey specks.
- Papular urticaria (small erythematous papules) at sites of feeding. Severe itching in pubic areas followed by feeding. Secondary changes of lichenification, excoriation.
- Secondary infections.
- **Maculae cerulae (taches bleues)** are slate grey or bluish grey macules 0.5 to 1 cm in diameter, irregular in shape, non-blanching. Pigment thought to be breakdown product of heme affected by louse saliva. Common on lower abdominal wall, buttocks, upper thighs.
- **Eyelash infestation:** Serous crust may be present along with lice and nits; occasionally, edema of eyelids with severe infestations.

MCQ

Distribution

Most common in pubic and axillary areas, also in perineum, thighs, lower legs, trunk especially periumbilical.

In hairy males: Nipple areas, upper arms, rarely wrists; rarely, beard and moustache area. Eyelashes and eyebrows may be infested.

Differential Diagnosis

Trichomycosis pubis, white piedra, scabies, mycosis.

Management

30% of persons with pubic lice have another concurrent STI, screen for them.

- 1% permethrin.
- GBHC 1% lotion.
- Malathion 0.5%.

Repeat treatment after 10 days.

MCQ

For eyelash/eyebrow involvement—Petroleum jelly or anticholinesterase eye ointment for 2 weeks.

SCABIES

Scabies is an infestation by the mite sarcoptes scabiei.

Synonym "7 years itch".

MCQ

Epidemiology and Etiology

- Scabies is essentially a disease of children. Among children the prevalence is highest in the age group below 5 years.
- Caused by *Sarcoptes scabiei* var hominis. The female mite is about 0.4 × 0.3 mm. They have **four pairs of legs.** The male is much smaller (0.2 × 0.15 mm).
- The female mite burrows though the stratum corneum and granular layer, at the rate of 2-3 mm daily. Usually burrow at night and lay eggs during the day. Female lives 4 to 6 weeks, laying 40 to 50 eggs (Fig. 3.4). The male mite dies after copulation. Usually in classic scabies there are about a **dozen females per patient (10-11 mites)** are present. In hyperkeratotic or crusted scabies, **> 1 million mites** may be present.
- Incidence at 300 million cases/year worldwide. In the past, epidemics occurred in cycles every 15 years.
- **Transmission:** Skin to skin contact, can also be sexually transmitted. Mites can remain alive for > 2 days on clothing or bedding; hence, scabies can be acquired without skin-to-skin contact.

Clinical Features

- Incubation period—often varies with immunity to the mite: First infestation, about 3 weeks, reinfestation, immediate i.e. 1-3 days.
- Itching characteristically described as 'worse at night', is the predominant symptom. Similar symptoms may be seen in several family members.

Two types of primary lesions are seen:

1. **Burrows: Pathognomonic** lesion of scabies. Gray or skin (Fig. 3.5) colored ridge 0.5-1 cm in length, either linear or wavy (serpiginous), with minute vesicle or papule at the end of tunnel. They are found in areas with few or no hair follicles, usually where stratum corneum is thin and soft, i.e. interdigital webs of hands > wrists> shaft of penis> elbows> feet> genitals> buttocks> axillae > elsewhere.
2. **Papules and Papulovesicles:** Due to hypersensitivity to the mite and appear as small erythematous papules or papulovesicles, which may be excoriated.

MCQ

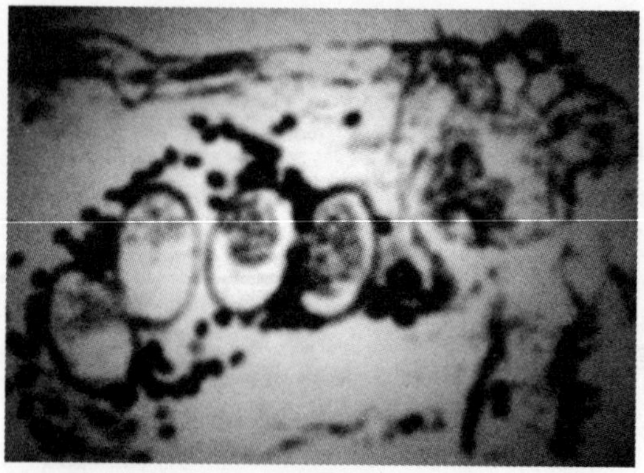

Fig. 3.4: Eggs, with scybala, with nymph (Scabies)

M C Q

• Specific (Treponemal) Tests

- Treponemal enzyme immunoassay (EIA) to detect IgG, IgG and IgM or IgM.
- *Treponema pallidum* haemagglutination assay (TPHA),
- *Treponema pallidum* particle agglutination assay (TPPA).
- Fluorescent treponemal antibody absorption test (FTA-ABS)
- *Request **EIA for anti-treponemal IgM*** if primary syphilis is suspected **IgM** is detectable towards the end of the **second week** of infection while **IgG** is detectable usually in the **fourth or fifth week**.

The majority of patients who have reactive treponemal tests will have reactive tests for the remainder of their lives, regard-less of treatment or disease activity. However, 15%-25% of patients treated during the primary stage revert to being serologically nonreactive after 2-3 years.

M C Q

• Cardiolipin (Non-treponemal) Tests

Venereal Diseases Research Laboratory (VDRL), Carbon antigen test/rapid plasma reagin test (RPR). A titer of > 1:8 is positive and it is the best test for **monitoring therapy**. A titre <1:8 is called False Positive VDRL.

M C Q

Interpretation

A *four fold* change in titer, equivalent to a change of two dilutions (e.g., from 1:4-1:16 or from 1:8-1:32), is considered necessary to demonstrate a clinically significant difference between two nontreponemal test results that were obtained using the same serologic test.

- **A VDRL/RPR titre of >1:**16 and/or a positive IgM test indicate active disease and the need for treatment, although serology must be interpreted in the light of the treatment history and clinical findings.
- For purposes of partner notification and presumptive treatment of exposed sex partners, patients with syphilis of unknown duration who **have high nontreponemal serologic test titers (i.e.,>1:32)** can be **assumed** to have early syphilis. However, serologic titers should not be used to differentiate early from late latent syphilis for the purpose of determining treatment.

Recommended for Screening

Treponemal EIA (preferably IgG and IgM) or TPPA or VDRL/RPR and TPHA.

M C Q

EVALUATION OF SEROLOGICAL TESTS

Confirmation of Infection: 2 Positive Tests with Specific Test.

Assessing Degree of Activity: IgM FTA-ABS and VDRL >1:64.

Second Infection: VDRL titre increase by two dilution and new appearance of IgM antibodies.

DIAGNOSIS OF NEUROSYPHILIS

Microscopy: lymphocytes > $5/mm^3$.
Biochemistry: protein > 0.4 gm/l.
Serology: VDRL (negative in > *1/4* neurosyphilis).
FTA or TPHA (negative test virtually excludes neurosyphilis).

Neurosyphilis is unlikely when the CSF TPHA *titre is < 1:320 or the TPPA titre <1:640.*

The TPHA index (CSF TPHA/albumin quotient [CSF albumin × 103/serum albumin]) allows for impaired barrier function and is more sensitive than the CSF VDRL whilst maintaining high specificity. M C Q

A TPHA index >70 and a CSF TPHA titre >320 are the most reliable in supporting a diagnosis of neurosyphilis but unfortunately determination of the TPHA index is not widely available.

DIAGNOSIS OF CONGENITAL SYPHILIS

M C Q

- *Direct demonstration* of *T. pallidum* by dark ground microscopy and/or PCR of exudates from suspicious lesions, or body fluids, e.g. nasal discharge.
- *Serological tests* should be performed on **infant's blood** not cord blood and if the infant's serum is positive on screening, perform treponemal IgM EIA, quantitative VDRL/RPR and quantitative TPPA tests on the infant and mother in **parallel**.
- **Serological tests detecting IgG** may be positive due **to passive transfer** of maternal antibodies whether or not the infant is infected.
  - If the IgM test is negative, and the other tests are reactive with titres less than four-fold higher than those of the mother and there are no signs of congenital syphilis, then repeat reactive tests at 3, 6 and 12 months of age or until all tests become negative (usually by 6 months). Also repeat the IgM at 3 months in case the infant's response is delayed or suppressed.
  - If the infant's serum is negative on screening, and there are no signs of congenital infection, no further testing is necessary.
- A positive **IgM EIA test** and/or a sustained **four fold or greater difference of VDRL/RPR titre or TPPA titre above that of the mother** (confirmed on testing a second specimen from the infant) indicates a diagnosis of congenital infection.

MCQ

Table 9.2: Antigen–Pemphigus

Variant	*Tissue antigens*
P. vulgaris	**Dsg 3, Dsg 1**, desmocollins, plakoglobin, cholinergic keratinocyte receptor (CKR- alpha9 and pemphaxin), annexins, α chain of high affinity IgE
P. vegetans	**Dsg 3, Dsg 1,** desmocollins 1 and 2
P. foliaceus	**Dsg1**,desmoplakin, periplakin, envoplakin, plakoglobin
P. herpetiformis	**Dsg 3, Dsg 1,** desmocollin
P. erythematosus	Dsg1(3),ANA, 230kDa, 190 kDa, periplakin
Drug-induced	heterogenous
IgA - SCPD type	**Desmocollins 1&2**
IgA - IEN type	**120 kDa, Dsg 1 & 3**
Atypical IgG/IgA	Desmocollins 1-3
Paraneoplastic	Envoplakin,periplakin,desmoplakin 1 & 2, BP-230,plectin, Dsg1&3,170 kDa transmembrane antigen
Endemic	Dsg 1, 3

MCQ

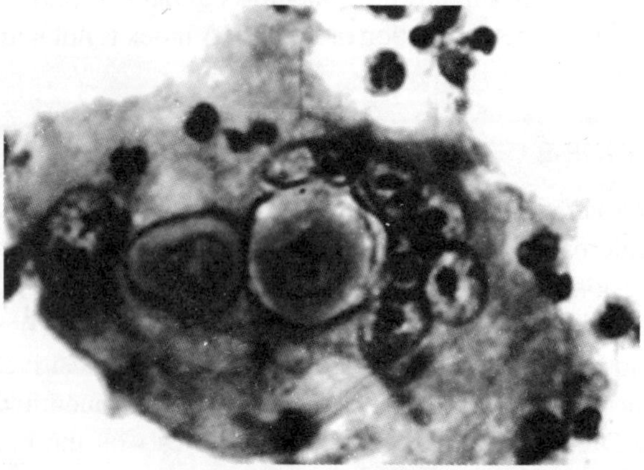

Fig. 9.3: Multiple acantholytic cells

MCQ

Clinical Features (Figs. 9.4(a) to 9.4(c))

Mucosal lesions are seen in almost all the patients. Either the onset is with painful oral erosions (50-70%) or is involved during the course of the disease. Other mucosae involved are conjunctiva, pharynx, larynx, oesophagus, urethra, vulva and cervix.

Skin lesions are asymptomatic, flaccid bullae on normal or erythematous skin. The sites involved are scalp, face, trunk, axillae and groins (flexural surfaces). Rupture of bulla causes painful erosions that heal spontaneously leaving behind hyperpigmented macules. Peeling of skin takes place when tangential force is applied **(Nikolsky's** sign). Bulla spread sign **(Asboe-Hansen sign)** is also positive.

Course and Complications

Prognosis is poor without treatment but with systemic steroids, mortality has been reduced to 5-15%.

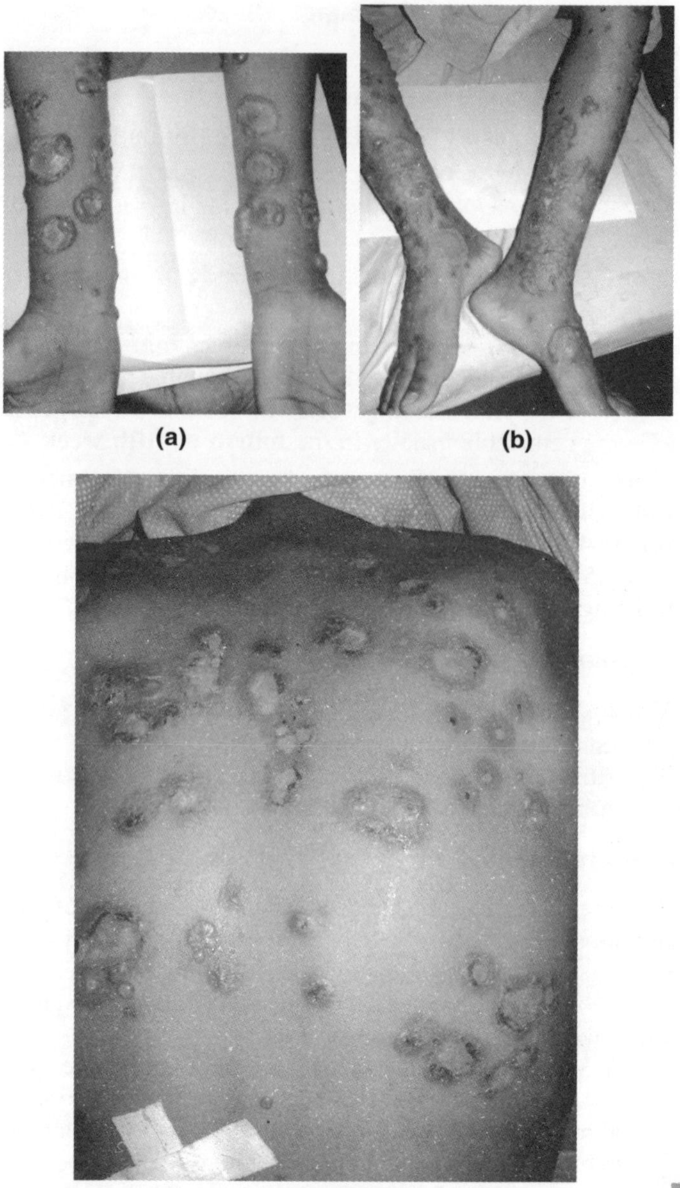

(a) (b)

(c)

Fig. 9.4(a) to 9.4(c): Multiple erosions and flaccid bulla on the back and extremities

Even with the use of corticosteroids and other immunosuppressive agents, there is still significant morbidity and mortality associated with pemphigus vulgaris. A common cause of death is infection secondary to the immunosuppression required to treat the disease. Most deaths occur within the first few years of the disease. Unfortunately, many of the drugs used to treat this disease have serious side effects, and patients must be monitored closely for infection, renal and liver function abnormalities, electrolyte disturbances, hypertension, diabetes, anemia, and gastrointestinal bleeding.

CHAPTER 9

VESICULOBULLOUS DISORDERS

The vesiculobullous diseases although uncommon have a social and economic impact on the patient and the family. These are classified into **genetic** (epidermolysis bullosa) and the **acquired autoimmune** blistering disorders (pemphigus, bullous pemphigoid, dermatitis herpetiformis, chronic bullous dermatosis of childhood, epidermolysis bullosa acquisita) (Table 9.1).

Table 9.1: Classification of disorders based on histopathological level

Intra-epidermal disorders	*Dermal-epidermal junction*
Granular layer	***Junctional (at the lamina lucida)***
• Friction blister	• Junctional epidermolysis bullosa
• Pemphigus foliaceus	• Bullous pemphigoid
• Subcorneal pustular dermatosis	***Dermolytic (below basal lamina)***
• Staphylococcal scalded skin syndrome	• Epidermolysis bullosa dystrophicans
• Bullous impetigo	• Epidermolysis bullosa acquisita
Spinous layer	• Porphyria cutanea tarda
• Eczematous dermatitis	• Dermatitis herpetiformis
• Herpes virus infection	
• Familial benign pemphigus	
Suprabasal	
• Pemphigus vulgaris	
• Darier's disease	
Basal layer	
• Erythema multiforme	
• Lupus erythematosus	
• Lichen planus	
• Epidermolysis bullosa simplex	

Intercellular-Adhesion Molecule (Fig. 9.1)

The intercellular adhesion, molecule between the keratinocytes is called cadherin. A detailed analysis reveals that the intercellular substances is composed of desmocollin and desmoglein and the component within the cell is composed primarily of desmoplakin and plakoglobin. Similarly the basement membrane zone is composed of numerous strectures (Fig. 9.2) that play a role in bullous disorders.

Classification of Pemphigus

- Pemphigus vulgaris
- Pemphigus foliaceus
- Pemphigus erythematosus (Senear Usher)
- Pemphigus vegetans (Neumann, Hallopeau)
- Fogo Selvagem: Endemic
- Drug-induced
- IgA (SCPD, Intra-epidermal type) pemphigus
- Paraneoplastic pemphigus

Pemphigus

Definition

Pemphigus, an autoimmune disease is characterized by intraepidermal blistering at various levels in the epidermis, because of disruption of the intercellular cementing substance. It is due to an autoantibody attack (IgG) on the cellular adhesion proteins (desmogleins) (Table 9.2) leading to acantholysis seen on tzanck smear (Fig. 9.3).

Epidemiology

Rare, equal in men and women, onset at 40 to 60 years of age, more common in Jewish or Mediterranean descendants.

Aetio-Pathogenesis

MCQ

Antibody **IgG1 and C3** against **DG 3** (Table 9.2).

Drugs: Sulfydryl group-penicillamine, captopril, rifampicin.

Others (beta blockers, cephalosporins, penicillin and rifampicin).

INVESTIGATION

Bedside Tests

***Grattage Test*:** When the psoriatic plaque is scraped with a glass slide, the very characteristic silvery scales come out that is known as the Candle Wax/Grease Sign.

***Auspitz Sign*:** The successive removal of psoriatic scales usually reveals an underlying smooth glossy red membrane (**Berkley membrane**) with small bleeding points which appear when the thin suprapapillary epithelium is torn off.

Histopathology (Fig. 11.9)

There is parakeratosis associated with focal orthokeratosis and **Munro's microabscess formation,** near absence of the granular layer, **spongiform pustules in the Malpighian layer**, hyperplasia with elongation of rete ridges and suprapapillary epidermal thinning, mononuclear leukocyte infiltrates in the lower half of epidermis.

Dilated, tortuous papillary blood vessels almost touch the undersurface of the thinning suprapapillary epidermis and are surrounded by a mixed mononuclear and neutrophil infiltrate, as well as extravasated erythrocytes.

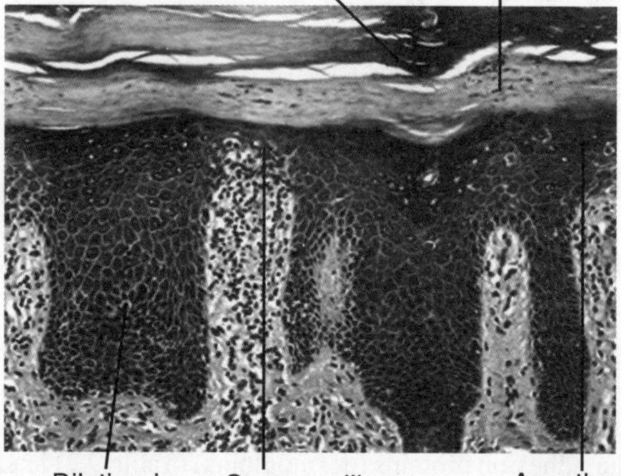

Fig. 11.9: Lymphocytes around vessels, thin rete ridges of about equal length, marked spongiosis and hyperkeratosis and parakeratosis

Treatment (Table 11.3)

Table 11.3. Treatment of choice for specific type of psoriasis

I. Plaque psoriasis or psoriasis vulgaris	Topical therapy remains the mainstay of treatment	
(a) *Less than 10% BSA* (Mild and Moderate)	1. Emollients 2. Coal tar cream 3. Vitamin D analogue	
(b) Severe plaque psoriasis or affecting ***10%-20% BSA***	1. **PUVA** 2. PUVAsol 3. Narrow band UVB	Plus topical +emollient
(c) **'Severe' psoriasis** affecting ***>20% BSA and/or PASI >12***	1. **Methotrexate** 2. Acitretin 3. Cyclosporine 4. Hydroxyurea	
II. **Erythrodermic psoriasis**	1. Methotrexate 2. Acitretin	
III. Pustular psoriasis **(a) Localized**	1. **Acitretin** 2. Methotrexate	
(b) Generalized	1. **Acitretin** 2. Methotrexate	
IV. Palmoplantar psoriasis	1. Topical PUVA / PUVAsol 2. Highly potent steroid and salicylic combination	
V. Psoriatic arthritis	1. Methotrexate 2. Acitretin	

Therapeutic Modalities

Many effective therapies are available for treatment of the various clinical forms of psoriasis; each is useful and may be the appropriate initial therapy in a given situation.

Topical Therapy

Numerous topical agents are available. Topical therapy alone offers excellent control for many localized forms of psoriasis.

1. **Bland emollients:** Liberal use of emollients to soften and hydrate the epidermis is a cornerstone of psoriasis therapy after soaking in warm water.
2. **Keratolytics:** These agents remove scale, soften plaques, and enhance penetration of other therapies, though they do not treat the inflammation of psoriasis. They are most effective when used after adequate hydration.
   a. Salicylic acid 2%–10% in petrolatum is applied twice daily and is allowed to remain on the lesions.
   b. Salicylic acid 6% gel, is particularly useful for hyperkeratotic lesions of palms and soles. Do not use salicylic acid on greater than 20% of the body surface area, and use caution with widespread occlusion to prevent salicylate toxicity.
3. **Topical steroids:** Topical steroids are optimally used in combination with nonsteroid agents to both increase efficacy and decrease side effects.

   Though these should be avoided in high-risk areas such as the face, groin, axillae, and other skin folds. Combination of topical steroids with calcipotriene, tazarotene, or both may increase efficacy, decrease steroid-induced atrophy, prevent irritation from the nonsteroid agents, and prevent rebound and tachyphylaxis when used sequentially.